MW01061387

# Sasha's Tail

# Sasha's Tail

## LESSONS FROM A LIFE WITH CATS

## Jacqueline Damian

W. W. Norton & Company

NEW YORK • LONDON

Copyright © 1995 by Jacqueline Damian

All rights reserved
Printed in the United States of America
First Edition

The text of this book is composed in 11/14 Caslon
with the display set in Berkeley Old Style
Composition and manufacturing by the Haddon Craftsmen, Inc.
Book design by Micheal Chesworth


ISBN 0-393-03731-2
W.W. Norton & Company, Inc., 500 Fifth Avenue, New York, N.Y. 10110
W.W. Norton & Company Ltd., 10 Coptic Street, London WC1A 1PU
1 2 3 4 5 6 7 8 9 0

*For my mother and father*

# Contents

"You can learn a lot about all cats by looking closely at one of them."

—Richard Preston,
in a *New Yorker* article on
mathematicians' search for pi

# *Preface – People with Tails*

This is a book about cats or, more specifically, about my cats, especially one of them, a black and white cat named Sasha who in my opinion exemplifies feline virtue despite a few character flaws.

Writing about Sasha, and through him cats in general, has been an interesting experience, and a much broader one than I first anticipated. Writing about cats plunges you into an existential thicket that keeps shifting ground, Birnam Wood to Dunsinane, the more you move around in the territory.

One of my friends, who has lived with both cats and dogs, calls these animals "people with tails." Another friend, who once had a white collie show dog and later an Airedale named

Gwendolyn who grew up with his sons, does not. "Animals are animals," he insists, a little crankily. "You can't view them like people, because they're not."

Somewhere in between these two poles sits Sasha.

Sasha often seems like "people with tails." He has opinions, which he does not hesitate to make known, likes and dislikes, joys and fears. He is an undeniably emotional being, given, as we humans are, to displays of affection, jealousy, dominance, playfulness, embarrassment, and aggression, among other things. Whether he is also a thinking being I do not know, although it could be argued that thinking and feeling are not discrete functions but inseparable ones, way stations along the continuum of sentience.

Yet Sasha is very much an animal, a four-legged creature who lacks language, creates no tools or artifacts, and lives by no discernible moral or ethical code except for whatever cosmic laws might govern the lives of cats. He hunts with a passionate intensity, unencumbered by guilt and betraying no signs of anything akin to remorse (indeed, quite the opposite). He is attuned to his own instinctual nature in a way that human beings—i.e., people without tails—are not.

Arguably, all animals possess consciousness of some sort—or anyway, all animals with a spinal column, which is where one school of biologists draws the line between "us" and "them." They know they're alive, and so they share some common ground with us in terms of how we all experience the world. (Given that the tail is an extension of the spine, calling cats "people with tails" doesn't seem so far-fetched from this angle.)

But cats and dogs are different. They parted company with the rest of their backboned brethren the moment they moved indoors and took up residency within the human circle. At that point—perhaps twenty thousand years ago for dogs and a mere four thousand or so for cats—these once-wild creatures entered the oxymoronic realm of what we call domesticated animals.

This is where the problem arises, from the human point of view. We really don't know how to see such creatures. Animals, yes, as my one friend insists, and not fur-bearing pseudo-people. But humanish, too, at least in some ways, as we discover when we live with them and attend to what they tell us. On one level, these animals are our "pets." On another, they are fellow travelers. For we humans are "domesticated animals" ourselves, albeit self-domesticated, grappling with our instincts and impulses—our own conflicted nature—as we learn to live in society with others, just like our cats and our dogs. The push and pull of nature and culture, impulse and restraint, work relentlessly upon us, as upon them. Freud didn't write *Civilization and Its Discontents* for nothing.

Cats are particularly fascinating companions on this journey because they are domesticated, but not fully. Perhaps it's because they've sat at the human hearth for only a few millennia, thousands of years less than dogs. Perhaps it's because they've never been bred, as dogs have, to do much of anything for man. Except for mousing—a task they're all too happy to take on with no prompting from us—cats don't work for a living. Or perhaps there's something in the very nature of the cat that defies domestication. For even the cuddliest puss, a major feline couch potato, has something in him of the lion. Anatomically and behaviorally, cats are astoundingly alike, wherever they live and whatever their size.

There's something eminently enjoyable for us cat owners in the idea of the lion in the house, for as card-carrying members of the fellowship called Western Civilization we're imbued with romantic notions about wilderness and its denizens, the wild ones. In these days of environmental Armageddon, the bald eagle and the spotted owl, the Bengal tiger and the African elephant are potent symbols of paradise (almost) lost.

Of the animals we live with we're a touch less elegiac. Coddle them we might, and yet, philosophically, we view them as something less, somehow, than the noble creatures of the wild. Perhaps familiarity really does breed contempt. It's as if cats and dogs lost a little of their luster, and the right to be taken wholly seriously, the moment they drew close to man. We assume, without thinking too much about it, that nature is Out There, sacred but distant; it's not where we live. Where we live is Civilization, that vaguely tainted place we inhabit with our domestic animals. The cat, who straddles both worlds, is a fascinating, mysterious anomaly.

But maybe there's a trail of breadcrumbs leading through this thicket. Maybe our cats have something to tell us about the struggle we both share: how best to reconcile nature and culture, autonomy and community, love and independence. Maybe Sasha is as fruitful a subject of study as George Schaller's pandas or Jane Goodall's chimps. This, at least, was my working hypothesis when I began jotting down observations of my cats.

*       *       *

Sasha is the perfect cat to start with, for he leads an exemplary life for a cat. Living in the country, he has one foot in the wild, as a cat should. But surrounded by humans, he is a house cat, too. *Felis catus* in all his ambiguous splendor, artfully breaching the dual universe that we ourselves inhabit.

He can be independent, sometimes irascible. And yet he is bound through both circumstance and affection in a rich, complex social life with the other two cats in the household, Charcoal and Tigger, and with me and the other humans in our circle. Observer and participant both, he is a whole other, vivid intelligence residing alongside me in my home.

Does that make Sasha "people with tails"—or is he something else altogether? Psychologists have yet to decide, although interest in understanding animal consciousness is growing. The question could use referral to Freud, but the great debunker himself remained silent on the subject of animals, perhaps in deference to his dogs, a series of red chows to whom he was uncommonly devoted.

The last of them, a female named Lun, shared the Freud family's flight from Nazi Vienna to England in 1938. Grainy, black and white home movies that once belonged to Anna Freud and are now on view at the Freud Museum in London show a jittery Lun ducking behind Sigmund Freud's legs and accepting a comforting pat on the head during a brief stopover in Paris, where Lun found Princess Marie Bonaparte's bigger and more aggressive chow intimidating.

Once in England, Lun was sent ignominiously off into quarantine, as British law demanded. Frail and ill with the palate cancer that would kill him less than a year later, the eighty-two-year-old Freud nonetheless made a tiring trip across London on the arm of his daughter, Anna, to visit his exiled pet. It was an act that could not fail to endear the founder of psychoanalysis to the dog-loving English, and a newspaper called *The Referee* covered this event in some detail. The paper interviewed the head of the quarantine kennels, a Mr. Kevin F. Quin, who reported that Lun "leapt to meet [Freud] at his approach, glad recognition in every posture." It was impossible to say "which was more delighted," Quin told *The Referee*'s reporter: the young red dog or the elderly white-bearded doctor.

The paper assured its readers that Lun was well cared for and happy enough in quarantine, and that she played with the other dogs in Quin's care out in his back garden. She was reunited with her family after the requisite six-month wait, an event likewise commemorated by the English press. Amid the other memorabilia on view at the Freud Museum is a yellowed newspaper clipping showing Lun with Anna Freud, both of them smiling broadly, on the day of the dog's release.

* * *

The museum archives do not record whether Freud ever had a cat. But it's easy to imagine him with one. (With her small, perky ears and leonine ruff, Lun even looks a little bit like a feline wannabe.) Cats, after all, have a lot in common with the classic Freudian analyst—seemingly aloof but in fact deeply involved with the humans who come under their purview. The patient, silent watchfulness of the cat could be likened to the analyst's evenly suspended attention—though cats will, in fact, tip their hands and reveal their judgments about us more often than analysts ever will.

I can picture a cat—a sleek, sand-colored Abyssinian, perhaps, descendant (some say) of the sacred cats of ancient Egypt—sitting attentively in Freud's dim, intricately appointed office amid the clutter of books and antiquities. The cat perches, Sphinx-like, atop the doctor's gleaming wooden desk, as artfully poised as the objects that crowd upon it—the bronze head of Osiris, the Egyptian god of the underworld, or the jade figure of a Chinese scholar that adorns an elaborately carved table screen. She sits there—for my imaginary Abyssinian is a "she"—alongside the doctor and listens with him to the dreams, fantasies, and free associations of Freud's analytic patients.

Here the metaphor wears thin, however, for the obverse of the meditative side of the cat's nature is a deepseated wish to be involved. Ask anyone who's ever had a cat. You can't wrap a present without an extended discussion with your cat about the proper use of ribbon (decoration or plaything?). You can't bring anything new into the house without your cat's exercising her right to thoroughly inspect it (all the better if the new thing comes in a paper bag or cardboard box, both of which cats find endlessly entertaining). You can't read a newspaper without your cat's attacking its pages—or watch TV without a cat-shaped silhouette in the middle of the screen. And you can't write without a cat stalking about your desk, tripping across your computer keyboard, and leaving wafts of hair behind to gum up the workings of the mouse.

Back in the office of Dr. Freud, my imaginary Aby would soon tire of her observer's role. She would look for some interesting item in Freud's formidable collection of art objects—an Egyptian scarab, perhaps, or a Japanese netsuke—to use as a toy, and send it clattering across the floor. She would bedevil the doctor as he tried to take notes by batting away at his fountain pen. She would leap from the desk to the famous Persian carpet–draped analytic couch, and curl up for a snooze atop the unsuspecting analysand.

◆　　◆　　◆

I bring to this project all the enthusiasm of a dedicated amateur, someone untrained in the disciplines of zoological fieldwork, but possessing a journalist's eye together with a deep and abiding interest in the supple creatures that have been a part of my life since I was a very little girl. Not long ago a friend asked me, only half-facetiously, "Have you ever met a cat you didn't like?" Truth to tell, I couldn't think of one.

As the future unfolds, I'll probably turn into one of those eccentric old ladies out of a Barbara Pym novel or a George Booth cartoon who keeps seventeen cats. In the meantime I have only three, and you are about to meet them in the pages that follow.

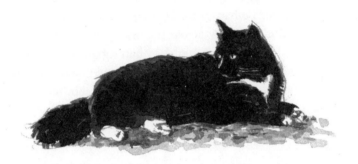

*W*hen an animal is taken from its environment, removed from its society and the harsh selection pressures to which it must accede, its character develops to a much greater degree than it would have in the wild. . . . A pet shows the inherent potential for individuality that lies largely dormant in a species.

—George B. Schaller,
*Golden Shadows, Flying Hooves*

# Sasha's Tail

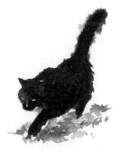

# 1  An Autobiography With Cats

I have always lived with cats. There are pictures of me in my grandparents' yard as a small child, certainly no more than three, wearing a sundress and a wide smile in the company of my mother and three little kittens. This would have been Eeny, Meeny, and Mo (there was no Miney), offspring of the inappropriately named Elmer, who was taken into our gray triple-decker house in Southbridge, Massachusetts, to deal with an invasion of mice.

Cantilevered into the hillside at the top of Cross Street, this big old house was home to a multigenerational Italian-American family. My mother and father and I lived in the apartment upstairs, my aunt and uncle and baby cousin, Karen, lived in the apartment downstairs, and my two teenage uncles lived with my grandparents in the main part of the house in the middle. We had two dogs: Wacky, a cheerful terrier mix who barked a lot; and Tappy, full name Tapioca Pudding, a tawny cocker spaniel my aunt had acquired on her honeymoon.

And then there was Elmer.

Elmer was a small gray tabby. We called her a "wildcat" because she never really got into the swing of living with humans. Valued as an efficient mouser, she was standoffish and distrustful of everyone except my mother, who, in retrospect, was probably the only human to pay her any mind. My grandmother certainly didn't. She was afraid of cats until the day she died, and never got used to ours.

One day Elmer disappeared, vanishing sylphlike into the woods, one hopes, as wild things must. But by then she had given birth to Meeny, who became our family cat.

A dainty tortoiseshell with a calligraphic "M" on her forehead and a gold, cream, and orange coat overlaid in pointillist black, Meeny kept us supplied with litter after litter of kittens over the years. When Meeny was young she had litters of three or four (even five, a couple of times), twice a year on average. As she matured, the litter size shrank to just one or two, and the frequency diminished as well. When she was very old—and she lived to be nineteen—she stopped having kittens altogether and relaxed in the pampered retirement she so richly deserved.

Meeny moved with us to a raw development of modest postwar ranches in West Warwick, Rhode Island—grandly named Windsor Park, as if it were royalty's playground—where my parents bought a light green house on a G.I. mortgage in 1952, the year after my brother was born. There she established herself as feline matriarch and, like her mother, Elmer, a mouser extraordinaire.

But this was the 1950s, prime time for Beaver and Ike, and

hardly anyone but us had a cat. Dogs were the animal of choice in the newly minted suburbs, and Meeny and her many kittens made our family stand out as, well, different. I'd like to say we gained distinction on their account, but in truth the neighbors seemed to find it just a little suspect, as if only beatniks, Communists, or unassimilated Europeans would be caught dead keeping cats. It didn't help that both my parents voted for Adlai Stevenson. Twice.

All through childhood my brother, Mike, and I got dragged into discussions with the other kids in the neighborhood over the relative merits of cats versus dogs. These arguments were a setup, though. No one bothered listening as Mike and I enumerated the virtues of cats. They were too busy banging the drum for dogs.

Dogs will save your life, said our friends. They will wake you up with their barking if a burglar breaks in while you're asleep. They'll drag you to safety if you fall through a hole in the ice—or pull a sled (Huskies), rescue skiers caught in an avalanche (St. Bernards), help firemen (Dalmatians), and guide the blind (Seeing Eye dogs).

None of us had ever known a dog this heroic, of course. Lady and Colonel and the other neighborhood mutts were goofy, irresponsible creatures whose idea of fun was to run away with the ball during our backyard softball games and return it to us, slimy with dog slobber, after an extended romp. Still, everyone knew that dogs could, and did, perform these feats, if they had to. Lassie and Rin Tin Tin celebrated such dogs on TV, and every once in a while the local paper would run a photo of some newsworthy canine hero, adding weight to the dog owners' arguments. These boiled down to one fact: dogs were utilitarian, whereas cats were not.

What could my brother and I say? We never told them that our kittens had a utility of their own—as performance artists.

*    *    *

What they performed was The Famous Trick, a regimen my father and brother and I imposed on generation after generation of kittens. Just when my father first dreamed up The Famous Trick—and moreover, why—I no longer recall. But once he did, it was tested on every litter that passed through the household.

Like a tennis coach with a child prodigy on his hands, Dad started the kittens off young. He began training when the litter of the moment reached that frisky stage—say, five or six weeks—the age when a kitten's ears are big and perky, its legs are coltishly long, and it looks more or less like a cat and not a baby seal, as it does when it's first born. This is an age of almost terrifying energy—a time when kittens whizz around like dust devils, leap stiff-leggedly into the air, bucking bronco-style, grab hold of their mother's ears (or human fingers) with pin-sharp teeth, and generally defy the notion that there is no such thing as perpetual motion. Whoever coined the phrase "weak as a kitten" must never have had one.

The Famous Trick went like this.

Kneeling on the living-room rug, Dad would corral a kitten by making a circle around it with his outstretched arms and barring it from leaving (as the kittens always tried to do by squirming through the gap between his upper arms and knees). Once incarcerated, the kitten quickly realized there was only one way out: by jumping. Aesthetics demanded that the leap be made at the centerpoint formed by my father's interlaced fingers and not, say, over his left forearm. So Dad would gently nudge the kitten into the midpoint of the circle and stroke its little chin upward, in order that it might peer over his hands and see freedom on the other side.

Up and over the little one would vault, to the cheers of the rest of the family, only to be snatched up again by my brother or me and coaxed to jump once more—this time a little higher. Dad would start the exercise with arms resting on the rug. As each kitten, in turn, began to master the basics of the trick, he gradually raised the circle of his arms a little bit more and a little bit more, so that their leaps became progressively elevated. A foot or so was pretty much the record, as I recall, but that's quite a jump for a young animal standing no more than six inches off the ground in its stocking feet.

Any kitten that tried to evade its responsibility by making a break for it via the low road—that is, by slipping underneath the symbolic barricade of Dad's arms—was ruthlessly tracked down by Mike and me and made to perform The Famous Trick again. This time, correctly.

We were, I should add, under no delusions that The Famous Trick represented anything more than the triumph of the cat's desire to regain autonomy and leap free of human interference. Actually, that was the joke. We liked our cats spunky, and unlike the dog owners, we didn't mind at all that they didn't do tricks—not real ones. Utilitarianism is an admirable thing in an animal, I suppose, but there's something refreshing, too, in its absence.

◆　　◆　　◆

Out of all of Meeny's kittens, there was one that I loved the most: Romeo, who was born, along with his sister, Juliet, when I was six or seven. I begged and begged to keep him. Meeny was the family cat, dubbed Beanhead—Bean, for short—by my brother as soon as Mike was old enough to talk. But I wanted a cat of my own, one who was all mine, and I wanted one so badly that finally my parents said Romeo could stay.

He was not what you would call a handsome cat. In fact, he was actually somewhat homely. Buff pink and off-white, he grew up to be a burly, big-headed tomcat sorely lacking the usual feline grace. I loved him all the more for that, reasoning that because he was less than beautiful no one else could possibly appreciate him the way I did. An unneutered male (we didn't know from neutering back in the fifties), Romeo roamed. Sometimes he stayed away for a couple of days, returning to gobble up large servings of Puss 'n' Boots cat food and laze around the house before setting off on further adventures. "Wherefore art thou Romeo?" took on new meaning for us.

Sometimes Romeo came home bloodied from catfights, in which he ultimately acquired notched ears and a scarred nose, like an aging pugilist. But I know he gave as good as he got, for I witnessed more than a few of these feline conflicts in or near our yard.

He ranged widely, and one time he came home covered from head to toe with soot. God knows where he had been; we didn't exactly live in an industrial district. We washed him in the kitchen sink with Breck shampoo. My brother and I cut up an old rain slicker to make four cat-size galoshes, which we fastened on Romeo's paws with fat rubber bands to keep him from scratching. My father held him down in the sink while my mother lathered and sprayed. I took a snapshot of this unusual event, which I still have.

For all of his street smarts Romeo was kind of awkward indoors, like a mountainman at a cotillion. For example, he never got used to the washing machine, which was in the kitchen, and skittered away in fear whenever my mother turned it on. Sometimes he careened smack into a wall in his haste to get away. By the time he got old he had lost most of his teeth, so instead of eating directly out of his dish he scooped up cat food with his right front paw and delivered it to his mouth like that. This never failed to amaze our visitors.

But he was my cat, and that was all that mattered. For years

I carried Romeo's picture around in my wallet, alongside snap-shots of my parents and brother and my own First Communion photo. He slept on my bed every night (or every night he was home), curling up by my chest or in the cat-size crook formed by my bent knees when I slept on my side, where he would purr and purr. I was acutely aware of his comfort, and shimmied over to one side of the bed to give him enough room to stretch. He was a mellow, good-natured soul, not unlike my cat Char-coal today, and more tolerant of my friends than children have any right to expect of a cat. He let us dress him up in dolls' clothes and ride him around in my toy carriage.

I was heartbroken to get back from Girl Scout camp the summer I was eleven and find that Romeo was snubbing me. Unsure, perhaps, of who I was after my week-long absence, he refused to sleep with me for the first night I was home. Instead, he stationed himself in the doorway to my room all night, and no matter how many times I hauled him up on the bed beside me, he jumped back down and resumed his place by the door.

This was my first lesson in life from a cat. Romeo was in-forming me that one's actions have consequences.

◆   ◆   ◆

Romeo notwithstanding, the cats I've been drawn to as an adult have been beautiful cats. It's hard, in fact, to find a cat that's not beautiful. Barn cat or show cat, they pretty much always look good. Legend has it that the prophet Muhammad took scissors to his own robe rather than risk disturbing his cat, Muessa, who was sleeping on it. It may be that the founder of Islam was demonstrating the necessity of showing some consideration for a fellow citizen of the planet. But it's just as likely that the sleeping cat made such a beautiful picture that Muhammad couldn't bear to disturb it.

Cats are ornamental—part living sculpture and part living

doll. Their smooth grace, supple form, and rippling muscula-
ture are a pleasure to watch, in action or at rest. Like dancers or
athletes, they rarely make a wrong or awkward move. Their
soft, rich fur, be it plushy or smooth, begs to be touched. Their
expressive eyes come in pellucid shades of amber, copper,
green, or blue, sometimes rimmed with black markings as emphatic as the kohl eyeliner of an Egyptian goddess, or of
Twiggy circa 1965.

Of the three male cats I live with today, Sasha is the most
debonair. A longhaired black and white—or tuxedo cat, in the
terminology used by my vet—he sports an elaborate white ruff
that rivals the artificial ones worn by prosperous Dutch burgh-
ers in seventeenth-century portraits. His paws are white, too.
Three have dainty scallops just above the toes where the white
fur meets the black; with no scallops to contain it, the white
creeps farther up the left rear leg, making that one paw look like
a lucky rabbit's foot.

Sasha's whiskers are a marvel, excessively long and curled at
the ends, like Salvador Dali's well-tended waxed mustache.
The white seems whiter than any white could be against the
inky black velvet of his face. Thinner, more delicate whiskers
are positioned above his eyes, like an old man's unruly eyebrows.

This is not to say that Sasha is a perfect specimen. He
wouldn't make best in show. His eyes are too close together and
very round, lending him the owlish look of a Kliban cartoon
cat, preternaturally wise and vaguely humanish. An upside-
down exclamation point, the kind the Spanish use, bisects his
nose, but because it's off-center, his face is asymmetric, almost
Cubist, as if Picasso had given the *Demoiselles d'Avignon* a cat.
A thin white chevron outlines his lower lip, and between upper
lip and nose is a tiny white mustache that looks painted on, like
Groucho's.

If I lavish more ink on Sasha than on my other two cats, it is through no fault of Charcoal's or Tigger's. Charcoal is a big, sleek panther with a broad nose, yellow eyes, and a dashing white blaze at his throat. And Tigger is a beautiful young ginger tabby with copper eyes that precisely match his fur. They can't help it if I happen to have a thing for longhairs.

I really don't know why. Romeo and Bean and the other cats we had when I was a little girl were domestic shorthairs, which is another way of saying no known breed and nothing special to recommend them, and I see a lot to admire in this low-maintenance variety of cat. But somehow, as an adult, I've gravitated to the wildly, impossibly furry kind—cats that demand grooming if they're not to be plagued with knots, even as they fight me when I get out the comb. (Sasha is a bear when it comes to combing, and is mollified only by cat treats at the end of the ordeal.)

The first of my longhaired cats was Melville, who looked a little bit like Sasha but with more white patches breaking up the black. He died young, and to comfort myself upon his passing I immediately laid claim to his sister Mimsy, also the kitten of a neighborhood cat called Mrs. Boots and her unknown husband, but a year younger. Mimsy was black, too, with a saucy white chin that made her look coquettish and a Dutch Masters ruff to rival Sasha's.

Then came Jean Arthur, part silver Persian, whose incredibly long fur was silky and fine as baby's hair. And now I have Sasha, who looks vastly bigger than his actual ten pounds simply on account of his fluff.

There's something so generous, so unstinting, about a longhaired cat. All that opulent fur—and for what? It's hard to see what advantage this abundance brings them, why natural selection, or whatever other laws govern the biological universe, found it necessary to create a niche for shaggy cats. Or maybe nature, to borrow from Mae West, had nothing to do with it; perhaps the fact that humans like them guaranteed fluffballs would flourish—a kind of assisted natural selection.

For Sasha, this elaborate do can be something of a burden. He comes home at least once or twice a summer with nettles embedded in his fur, a problem Charcoal and Tigger never face, and both he and I must work long and hard to get them out. Hairballs are another fact of life for many longhairs, the inevitable result of ingesting, during grooming, more fluff than the feline digestive tract can handle. As for protection from the cold, Sasha is more willing to venture outdoors in winter than Charcoal is, it's true, but less willing than Tigger, who likes to play in the snow. Go figure.

One advantage longhaired cats do have, though, is presence. A longhaired cat has Attitude, they know how to make a statement just by being there. They must learn it early, like natural blondes and Frenchwomen. And they're a sight to behold when aroused, by a passing dog or some other source of fright, to put up their backs Halloween-style. With hair standing on end, a longhaired cat resembles a porcupine *erectus* and looks a great deal bigger than he really is, which is the point. A dog might think twice before attacking a creature as large and imposing as this.

❖    ❖    ❖

Of the four longhairs I have had, the most elegant by far was Mimsy. Even as a kitten she had an inborn hauteur, a sense of herself as someone apart, someone blessed by nature and bearing all the responsibility of anyone so chosen. Her white whiskers were even longer than Sasha's are. Her big double paws, also white, gave the appearance of gloved hands, complete with opposable thumbs. Her fur was so thick and shaggy that she sometimes made me think of a yak. And since her nose was fairly long, as feline noses go, she always appeared to be looking down it, grande dame–style.

Mimsy had a favored posture when reclining that I've never seen another cat duplicate. Instead of tucking away all her limbs to form the neat, brisket-style package of other cats, she extended her two front legs and crossed them in front of her, one atop the other, like a pinup girl crossing her gams. When seated in this position, Mimsy also arched her head and torso slightly backward, away from her paws, which served to display her legs at their full extension.

It didn't take much imagination to see her as the Black Swan queen in *Swan Lake,* who in a famous solo speaks volumes with the eloquently stylized crossing and uncrossing of her arms.

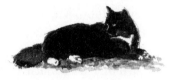

# 2 Love at the Cat-Food Counter

One of the TV magazine shows recently aired an episode about the pet-food industry that contained an intriguing nugget of information. It seems that the marketing geniuses at Ralston-Purina, Kal Kan, et al. operate on the assumption that there is a distinct difference between cat owners and owners of dogs.

The rule of thumb for these experts as they map out their advertising campaigns is that dog owners are sublimely confident of their dogs' loyalty and affection. Dogs are pals, members of the family, good old boys. You can always count on your dog.

Cat owners, on the other hand, are assumed to be gripped with something akin to existential angst. Cat owners, the marketing gurus believe, fear that their cats will reject them, and they buy cat food with all the trepidation of someone making that first romantic dinner for a new lover. (Does he like Italian food? I hope he's not allergic to tomatoes.) The finicky Morris and the pampered darlings of the Fancy Feast commercials, elegantly nibbling their canned victuals out of leaded-crystal goblets, are the perfect corporate spokescats. Yes, they will eat the food you put before them—but only if it's the *right food.* Otherwise they will vex and humiliate you by walking away from their bowls in a snit, and no amount of persuasion, much less coercion, will ever get them to change their minds.

This theory may be a teeny bit overdrawn, but as a cat owner of long standing I've got to admit it contains a grain of truth. Some cats are, in fact, terribly fussy, and it's easy enough to start believing their constant rejection of your offerings of food is also a rejection of you. Food is love, as a friend of mine is fond of saying.

My own cats, thank goodness, are not that way, but even these three omnivores have been known to turn up their noses at one thing or another from time to time. There are some types of cat food that they simply will not eat—or worse, that one or two of them will eat but the other one (or two) won't touch. Let's see, was it Savory Chicken that Sasha walked away from last week, or Chicken Hearts and Liver? Charcoal likes Seafood Supper but spurns Captain's Table, while Tigger prefers Alpo to Nine Lives—or is it the other way around?

Each week at the supermarket I join the other cat owners purposefully picking and choosing among the multifarious cans and boxes of dry, wet, and "semimoist" cat food. The latter has the shape and texture of flattened Raisinets and comes neatly packaged in little sealed pouches, each one the proper serving size, like those individually boxed breakfast cereals you get in a restaurant. Convenience food for cats.

Fish, meat, chicken, dairy. Food for kittens, food for special dietary needs, food for the golden-agers (Friskies Senior, Purina Cat Chow Mature). My memory often fails me when it comes to the particulars of who likes what, and choosing a brand the cats have never tried before can be cause for concern. Should I or shouldn't I? Will they like it, or will I have to throw it out? This is especially true of no-name house brands, about which I have the same feeling as someone buying a fake Gucci handbag from a street peddler. It looks like a Gucci, it smells like a Gucci, it feels like a Gucci—but in the depths of my cats' being, I fear, they will know it is ersatz and remind me that they deserve nothing so second-rate.

Sometimes we cat people share our burdens at the cat-food counter. "He won't eat anything but Friskies Beef and Liver," a fellow shopper confided not long ago. "She likes those horrible mackerel chunks in jelly. Ugh!" confessed another on a different day.

One time I watched a domestic drama unfold in front of the canned foods as an elderly woman turned thumbs down on every one of her husband's cat-food choices. Obviously, he just didn't know their cat's tastes as well as his wife did, and I got the feeling this lapse was merely the latest in a long string of disappointments he had caused her.

"She won't eat that one," the woman snapped, peering over her eyeglasses to scan the label on the can her husband handed her. Showing no sign of impatience, this meek, white-haired man put the can back on the shelf and picked out another one, only to be admonished, "No, no, she doesn't like sardines."

How inept he must have felt. And how he must have envied the dog owners up the aisle heedlessly hefting a sack of Dog Chow or a six-pack of Cadillac into their shopping carts and going cheerfully on their way.

❖    ❖    ❖

No question about it. Once you get a cat you've set yourself up for an ongoing dialogue with a whole other individuality—a willful, sometimes adversarial companion whose taste in cat food is just one of the things you will learn to take into account as the two of you begin cohabiting. A tiny ball of fluff your kitten or cat may be, and yet you can't help but notice that he is a certain particular Someone: a Cat, self-possessed, self-assured, a creature to reckon with. One who would sing, with Walt Whitman, the *Song of Myself.*

A cat doesn't have much say in the big decisions of the household in which he lives—you might decide to move, for example, without consulting him first. But he makes his presence felt in the small events of the day, in all their splendid multiplicity. Cats possess an uncanny ability to get what they want, or do what they like, even when opposed. It's the genius of *Felis catus* that domestication has not produced enslavement. But it's aggravating, too.

"I didn't want Martha to go outside," reports Claudette, "but she outwitted me and slipped through my legs when I opened up the door."

"I gave Sam his pill but he spat it out when I wasn't looking," Lisa laments.

"I had to take Ralph to the vet's," says my mother, "but he scampered outside when he saw me getting out the cat carrier and refused to come back until office hours were over. He's too smart for his own good."

In my household, Sasha is the most insistent of the three cats about getting his way, as befits the alpha male. Some call him snooty—presumptuous, even—but the way I see it, he's simply enjoying the perks that accrue with status. Charcoal, the number-two cat, is the most easygoing, while Tigger, the youngest, falls somewhere in between. He's just over a year and a half old, so Tigger's character is still being formed; I have hopes for his potential as a lap cat, something the other two, for the most part, are not.

Still, I can't count on any of them to do what I want, when I want, if ever.

Sometimes they will come for a cuddle when I request it, sometimes they will not. Sometimes they let me hold them, sometimes they struggle to get out of my arms. (Cats are good at this, and the fact that we are so much bigger and stronger than they are gives us scant advantage. Just try holding on to a cat that doesn't want to be held.) Sometimes they come scampering home when I stand at the door and call; other times, no.

If they can be a nuisance by making themselves scarce, at times they are too much with us. Sometimes one or another of my cats will jump on the dining-room table in the middle of dinner and casually stalk about sniffing everybody's plates, looking up at me in seeming incomprehension when I say, "Down!" or, "No!" Cats understand "No!" but they do not like it; physical removal and abundant apologies to your guests are the only recourse.

Sometimes they stare, and frequently they stare at you. It's not unusual for a cat to eyeball a person with a bold, unblinking gaze, and while some people find it flattering to be the object of such unswerving attention, others do not. The steady, intelligent feline gaze always seems to carry a hint of evaluation. What are cats thinking when they look at us that way? Depending on one's level of insecurity, it's not hard to imagine them proclaiming, like the handwriting on the wall, "You have been weighed in the balance and found wanting."

Actually, though, evaluation is not identical with judgment, or anyway with negative judgment, and I think cats stare at us simply because they find us interesting. In the wild, they must be preternaturally observant to be the successful hunters that they are. And they're equally watchful at home, where their livelihood depends not on the behavior of rodents or birds but on the actions of human beings. Cats are acutely attuned to moods and rhythms and changes in the emotional weather. On top of that, they're just plain nosy—the cat's intense curiosity is no myth. They've got to know what's going on, feel compelled to check out the scene and investigate anything unfamiliar—a new piece of furniture, for example, or the paper bag your groceries came in. It's a way of mastering the environment, of being a part of things, and not estranged.

When I brought home my prized antique cupboard not long ago—a circa 1865 country piece of satiny, butterscotch pine—Sasha was so much underfoot that he made it difficult for my friends and me to move the thing into place. He sniffed and scrutinized this fascinating new object, repeatedly rubbing up against it to mark it with his scent (and thus defuse its strangeness, and make it "his"). He climbed inside when we opened up the doors, the better to test out all the shelves, and finally, when the cupboard was in place against the wall, he leaped from the dining-room table into its recessed top and nosed around up there. All before we ever managed to set one bowl or dish inside.

It's a good thing we cat owners learn to live with—or even appreciate—such independence, for it's central to life with cats. Cats have a mind of their own. Their needs and wants and preferences are not to go unheeded. Their autonomy must always be respected, their curiosity satisfied. And if they demand Friskies Beef and Liver exclusively, well, then, so be it.

◆  ◆  ◆

I've lived with cats so long that I tend to take their contrarian nature for granted. It's just part of what is, like air. But a friend who just got his first kitten doesn't quite know what to make of her. This little beige tiger, rescued off the street at roughly three weeks old, gives him mixed messages.

"If I've been away," says my friend, "the cat is so ecstatic to see me that she throws herself at my feet, rolls around on her back, waves her paws in the air, and chirps. But once I've been home for a while, she ignores me. She runs around and plays, and won't have anything to do with me—unless *she's* in the mood, of course."

This kitten has deeply bonded with my friend, who had to feed her with an eyedropper when he first brought her home because she was too little to know how to eat or drink on her own. It's not indifference, or lack of love, that causes her to scamper off when he makes a grab for her. It's something deep in the nature of the beast.

Perhaps the crux of the matter lies in the symbol of the straight line. This is a geometry, as Vicki Hearne points out in her book *Adam's Task: Calling Animals by Name,* that cats seem to scorn. Just as there are no straight lines in nature, so there are none in a cat's world.

Consider, for example, Sasha's typical trajectory when he comes inside for dinner: In the front door with a diagonal swing over to the telephone stand, which he rubs with his right cheek to mark proprietarily, via glands near the mouth and on the forehead, with scent too subtle for human detection; a leap onto the counter that separates kitchen from living room, followed by a leap onto the antique pie safe opposite it and another to the kitchen workstation where I am scooping out the cat food. Then down to his food dish to eat.

This route is not the shortest distance between two points. It lacks Euclidean elegance, is needlessly convoluted, unless one subscribes to the ancient Chinese belief that devils fly in straight lines.

Similarly, when I stood at the front door tonight and called for Sasha to come in, he didn't make a beeline for home. Rather, he sprinted toward me down the gravel path in front of the house, skidded to a stop midway to sniff at a patch of grass that caught his attention, then raced forward again—and again stopped short to investigate something else. Finally he crossed through the garden, angled over to the fieldstone walkway leading to the door, and marched inside.

I stood there and waited, since I know from experience that if I should hie over and pick the cat up intending to carry him inside, he would struggle out of my arms and stalk regally toward the door, flicking his bushy black tail expressively to signal his annoyance.

If cats are sometimes mystifying, it's because they prefer the indirect to the direct, the oblique to the straightforward, the parabola to the straight line. It's as if, in bringing cats into our homes, we are introduced to a culture as intricate and riddled with taboos as any described in the anthropology texts—and where it's just as easy to give offense.

Say I am sitting on the couch reading or watching TV and Sasha wants to cuddle up with me. Never, ever will he leap directly onto my lap. First he walks back and forth in front of the couch and jumps on and off the coffee table a few times until he is sure he has my attention, staring at me intently all the while. After a moment, I catch on to the fact that I am being given my cue. I'm supposed to lie down on the couch, flat on my back (Sasha doesn't like being a lap cat; he prefers a reclining human), and drape the woolen throw that hangs from the arm of the couch over my chest and stomach. Then and only then will Sasha jump on me and begin the intensive front-paw kneading that precedes his settling down for a snooze. (Does he insist on the throw to protect me from his claws as he kneads?)

If I make a grab for him before the ritual backing and forthing has been fully played out, he squirms away and repeats the whole ceremony, circling around, jumping on and off the coffee table, and staring, this time with a hint of reproach in his eyes. Clearly, the decision to cuddle, and its timing, must be his and his alone; I cannot impose it on him or hurry it along.

Sometimes my untoward attempt at direct action so offends him that he ostentatiously marches to the front door as if he wants to go outside, casting a meaningful glance back over his shoulder. Since I know he does not, in fact, want to go out but wants instead to cuddle, I am chastened into lying down again, shawl in place, and passively awaiting his decision to circle in for another approach. Having made his point, he soon does.

❖    ❖    ❖

Perhaps these regular shows of recalcitrance represent not willfulness but lessons that are genetically programmed. Cats, after all, would not be the evolutionary success story they are if they had not assimilated caution.

Consider, for example, the stop-and-start route that Sasha takes when I call him to come home at night. It's not devised to vex me or to vaunt his independence, but simply to check up on his territory, using the nose to gather information about what's been going on and who's been passing through. A sensible precaution for a territorial animal.

By circling around and making sure I'm passive and prepared before he climbs on top of me for a nap, Sasha might be using the same circuitous moves he relies on when he stalks another prize, prey—or the same observational skills he uses in assessing any new situation. Also prudent, if you don't like nasty surprises.

And backing off when I make a sudden grab for him—well, maybe that's acknowledgment that I'm a bigger, more fearsome predator than he is, one with the potential to harm him if I so choose. (Since I hate being reminded of my own brute nature, I'm offended when my cat darts away. It's unflattering, after all, to be treated as if you're bent on felinicide.)

Once I lie down, Sasha has succeeded in cutting me down to size, so to speak. No longer do I tower above him. In fact, from Sasha's point of view I've assumed the submissive posture—belly-up and immobile. Our power is now more equitable, and we lie there contentedly, nose to nose, for a nap.

As for cat food, who can say? I used to think the cats had good reasons for turning down the cat food they turned down, and that I should respect their judgment in terms of brands and flavors. After all, I don't have to eat the stuff, they do. However, the theory doesn't seem to hold water, for a type of cat food they gobble up today might get left in the bowl to molder if I serve it again next week.

Maybe there's a statement here that transcends biology. Maybe the duet at the food dish—the continual wrangling between cat and human over flavor and brand, the purchasing instructions handed out, heeded, forgotten—is another reminder, should we still be needing one, that a cat cannot be shaped to our will. This sometimes intractable creature is someone we can love but never control. A cat comes to us on his own terms, but cannot be forced. Companion and housemate he may be; possession or plaything he is not.

And if our lesson resides in Friskies Beef and Liver, then, as I say, so be it.

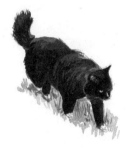

# 3  A Boy Named Sue

When visiting a friend in the hospital a while ago, I found myself distracted by the voices of the nurses in the hallway. "Where's Sasha?" one of them was asking. "Go find Sasha," murmured another. "Sasha . . . Sasha . . ." The sibilant sound seemed to echo in the corridors, and when the delinquent Sasha finally showed up, he turned out to be a burly, good-looking male nurse. Finally! I thought. A role model for my cat outside the realm of Russian literature.

I'm afraid I burdened Sasha with an existential problem when I gave him his name—not that he seems to mind, or even to notice, the gender confusion that swirls around him as if he were the Boy Named Sue. When I first brought him home, I thought he was a female. It's not that I don't know the difference. But with all that fluff making wispy pantaloons of his rear quarters, who could tell?

When Sasha subsequently revealed the truth of the matter, it was too late. He already knew his name. And, I don't know, he just seemed like a Sasha to me. I took refuge in the Russians, telling anyone who mistakenly called him "her" (people still do) that this Sasha was a veritable Alexander—as masculine as any count out of Tolstoy, or the Sasha at Roosevelt Hospital in New York.

The androgynous name is one of the things that Sasha and I both share. Until Jacqueline Kennedy stepped into the public eye in the early 1960s, I was the only female Jackie I knew, and all through childhood I was teased about my name.

"Jackie is a boy's name," my tormenters would say, pointing to the goodly supply of male Jackies in our neighborhood as proof. Even my own grandfather—my father's father, this is, not the Grandpa we lived with when I was small—sometimes got mixed up. We didn't see him that often, and he had at least seventeen other grandchildren to keep track of besides me. Still, it was galling whenever he greeted my brother, Mike, with a hearty "Hi, Jackie!" and then paused awkwardly, stuttering, "Hi, unh . . . unh . . ." when he turned his attention to me.

Never mind that it was his son, my father, who vetoed my mother's suggestions of Susan and Linda to name me for Jacqueline Cochran, the gorgeous blonde 1930s racing pilot. A contemporary of Amelia Earhart who dressed, Dietrich-like, in beautifully cut man-tailored suits, she went on to found the WASP (Women's Airforce Service Pilots) program during World War II and after the war became the first woman to break the sound barrier. As a radio operator on a B-17, and a man who loved flying, my father considered her a heroine. I often wonder what he had in mind in giving me her name.

＊　　＊　　＊

As for Sasha, he remained unnamed for a week or so after I found him. A friend and I kept trying names on him for size, hoping to find the one that suited him best. Finally I piped up with "Sasha!" and all three of us—two humans, one cat—seemed satisfied. The previous suggestion was Meatball, in honor of a crucial ingredient in the story of how I found him.

I first set eyes on this cat just about nine years ago. It was mid-October, and there was a chill in the air that dark Friday night as an old boyfriend and I made our way from my grandmother's house in Massachusetts to my mother's place in Rhode Island. We hadn't eaten, so we decided to stop at a little Italian restaurant—the kind with paper plates and red-checkered plastic on the tables—in a group of shops off a rural stretch of road in Scituate, Rhode Island. We climbed the rough wooden steps to the walkway connecting the stores, only to find ourselves face to face with a small but self-assured black and white cat.

He sat upright on his haunches and fixed us with the wise, attentive gaze I would come to know well in the years that followed. (The ancient Egyptian word for cat, *mau*, also meant "to see," which is apt. Cats do stare, even if you're not always sure at what.) Even in the shadows you could see he was a handsome creature: a half-grown kitten, perhaps five or six months old, with a long, fluffy tail and an endearing white smooch on his nose. We stopped to pet him, of course—Sasha is one of those cats that seem to invite caresses—and then went inside to order.

When I came back out five minutes later to phone my mother and tell her I'd be late, there was Sasha, waiting at the door. He trotted behind me to the phone booth and rubbed sweetly around my ankles all the time I was talking, in an apparent attempt (successful, in the end) to insinuate himself in my affections. After I hung up he followed me back to the restaurant, and he looked very disappointed indeed when I closed the door in his face.

But Sasha is not one to be easily deterred. In a moment the door opened again as new customers came in, and Sasha hurtled in along with them. Blinking broadly for a moment as his eyes adjusted to the light, he scanned the restaurant until he spotted my companion and me. He then marched directly to our table.

By this time the two of us had begun discussing whether we should take the cat home. He was bewitching us, all right. But he didn't have the hallmarks of a stray—too clean and friendly, seemingly healthy, and apparently well fed. He must, I said, already have a home.

"Oh, no," replied our waitress, who materialized like a *deus ex machina* at just this critical moment. "That cat used to live at the house up the road, but the people there kept the mother and kicked out the kittens. He's been living out of our dumpster for a while now."

I chopped up one of my meatballs and put it on a plate to bring outdoors for the cat—who, the waitress said firmly, was not allowed to stay inside—and thought about what to do. At the time I already had two cats, and I knew the last thing these thirteen-year-old females wanted was a kitten in the house to harass them. They had protested in no uncertain terms the one time I brought home a stray, but luckily for all of us that obliging little calico seduced the electrician who was rewiring my kitchen at the time, and went happily home with him.

I picked up Sasha, took him and the meatball outside, and went back in to finish my meal and consider my options. No, I decided. Cute as he was, I couldn't take him home. I did not need another cat.

But when my companion and I left the restaurant a little while later, there was Sasha, waiting by the door. He had finished the meatball and looked up at us expectantly. What could be said in the face of the inevitable? My friend and I looked wordlessly at each other and opened the car doors as Sasha made his way down the stairs, pausing for a moment midway as if to ponder his future. He glanced back over his shoulder at the restaurant that had been his erstwhile home, then craned his neck to peer into the car. He looked back again, and again peeked into the car. Apparently having settled the matter to his own satisfaction, he jumped inside, climbed on my lap, and leaned hard against me in a kind of armless hug. He gave me a long, lovestruck look, heaved a big sigh, circled around in my lap, and settled down to sleep. The redoubtable Sasha had found himself a home.

*     *     *

There seem to be two schools of thought about how to name a cat. One school uses people names, like Sasha. Sometimes these are old-fashioned or archaic people names, like Melville and Mimsy; or famous-people names—like Jean Arthur—that are silly (but cute) when applied to a cat. The other school uses names you would never give a human unless you were deranged. Charcoal and Tigger, for example.

As you can see, I fit both categories.

Melville was named after Herman. His sister Mimsy was named after Miriam, the friend who owned their mother, Mrs. Boots. The *Jabberwocky* allusion—in the line "All mimsy were the borogoves"—was serendipitous.

Jean Arthur started off as Arthur, after Arthur, Illinois, which is where I found her shortly after my former husband and I moved to that state. When she turned out not to be a male—a reverse foreshadowing of Sasha—there was nothing to do but call her Jean Arthur, after the smart blonde sidekick of countless 1930s comedies.

Charcoal was named for his color, which is black, by a little girl of my acquaintance. The word usually modifies gray, but take a look at a new piece of charcoal the next time you set up the grill; Anna was 100 percent correct.

And Tigger, of course, is named for the tiger in A. A. Milne's *Winnie the Pooh*, whom he resembles. I've since come to wonder if I shouldn't have found a more distinctive moniker for him. My old friend John used to complain that his name was too common—"Every Tom, Dick, and Harry is named John," he would say—and the same could be said about Tigger. Many, many people have told me they too have a cat named Tigger, or used to have a cat named Tigger, or know someone with a cat named Tigger. Not all of these Tiggers are tigers, either. At least one of them is black.

Naming is the first step toward relationship, for we name something only in order to know it. Sarah, a child I know in rural Maine, named each and every one of the lambs born one year at her family's farm Sarah, in honor of herself. More democratically, my friend Ann, maiden name Mason, christened the family cat of her childhood Mase, signaling that he too was a bona fide member of the clan. At the other end of the subject-object scale is a friend in Vermont who named her kitten Heineken, after the beer bottles that were the most salient feature of the house where the cat was living when she got her.

It may or may not be true that those who give their cats "people" names identify with them more closely than those who do not. Personally, I don't know if I could warm up to a cat named Heineken—although Charcoal bears the name of an inanimate object, and I don't have a problem with him. Maybe it's just that I don't like beer. On the other hand, I don't know if I could warm up to a cat named, say, Stalin—not that I know one, thank goodness (though I do know a black cat named Satan). Perhaps it's not a question of a people name but of a name that resonates emotionally, in a positive way, for the namer.

Now, Eeny, Meeny, and Mo—those were rather cold names my maternal grandparents gave to their cat Elmer's three kittens. You might as well name them One, Two, and Three (actually One, Two, and Four, given the absence of a Miney) as to call them Eeny, Meeny, and Mo. The names bespeak little affect, which, in retrospect, probably reflected Grandma and Grandpa's world view. These cats were mousers, not members of the family.

Meeny moved up the Scale of Being once she joined my nuclear family—especially after my brother came along and rechristened her Beanhead, in what must have been a juvenile stab at Cockney rhyming slang. Indeed, it's fun to riff on your cat's name, the way the obnoxious guy at the Xerox machine plays with his colleagues' names in those *Saturday Night Live* skits. The results can be telling.

For example, Sasha is always just Sasha to me, as if, like God, he's above being nicknamed. (Okay, I'll admit that once in a while I call him Mr. Fuff.) Charcoal, on the other hand, has a slew of aliases, including Charc-Man, the Charcmeister, Charky Coalcat, Chaka Khan, and just plain Charks. Tigger gets the baby names—Tiggy-pooch, Tigster, and Little Tigg Man, in honor of the old Dustin Hoffman movie—although lately I've been calling him plain old Tigg, in unconscious deference, perhaps, to the fact that he's suddenly grown to humongous proportions and outweighs Sasha now. Sometimes I call him Tigg Tigg Tigger, which I like because it reminds me of T. S. Eliot's Rum Tum Tugger.

Since Beanhead had so many kittens, naming them was a constant preoccupation for my brother and me growing up. We went through a literary period, from whence came Romeo—a perfect name for one's first (feline) love. We had Heckle and Jeckle, who were as peripatetic as the fast-talking cartoon magpies they were named for, and like them did everything together—including climbing the living-room drapes, one on either panel. The kitten we called Jack "S," a name borrowed from the *Li'l Abner* comic strip, turned out to be as stubborn as a jackass about using a sand box (the only kitten I ever remember who couldn't or wouldn't be trained).

But not every cat took on the character suggested by its name. Machiavelli, the black and white Persian my parents got after Beanhead died, bore no resemblance to the great manipulator of Renaissance Florence. She was ditsy, and looked a lot like Felix.

❖   ❖   ❖

There's a kind of rough poetry in naming. I have known a black cat named Midnight, a tuxedo cat named Skonk, a calico named Mudpie who looks like she has a dirty face, and a cat who was called Racer for the white stripe that ran down her forehead: it reminded my brother of a racing stripe on a car. Dusty is dust-colored, Rusty is rust-colored, and Houdini disappears. There's Sophie and Emma (named by a Jane Austen fanatic), Nigel and Martha, Argyle and Pip ("We have Great Expectations for him," his owners say). There's Bear and Roo—so named because she sits up on her haunches like a kangaroo—and two each of Charlotte and Max. There's Perkins, who's perky, and Itty Bitty Kitty, who's small. My cousin's cat is Ramada, because they found her at a Ramada Inn, and my aunt has Dirty Harry, a Himalayan named for the sorry sartorial state he was in when she got him.

Our county library holds an outdoor sale every spring and fall, setting up across its sweeping lawns table after table heaped with used (or "pre-owned") books. At the last one I picked up a hardcover copy of *Dreamgirl: My Life as a Supreme,* by Mary Wilson, and opened it to find on the inside back cover a list, neatly block-printed in black ink, of the names of eighteen cats. This was followed by the notation "plus 14 kittens." Six cats had death dates after their names, as in a newspaper obituary.

"Since 9/1971 32 cats have taken up residence in my home & heart," wrote the person who owned the book before me, adding that only two remained. For the record, the cats were Biddle, Sweetpea, Annie Orphan, Snow White, Puffy, Kitten, Whisper, Dinah, Babykins, Calli, Smokey, Whacky, Blacky, Tiggi-Wooger, Lulu, Six-Toe, Cutsie, and Little Guy.

I imagine Snow White, Smokey, and Blacky were named for their color; perhaps Calli was, too—it might be short for Calico. Six-Toe must have been a polydactyl, as double-pawed cats are properly called. Annie Orphan no doubt was a stray, and Puffy perhaps was a longhair. Personally, I like Dinah best; that was the name of Alice's cat in the Wonderland books. But wait a minute. Tiggi-Wooger? I think I'll try that one out at home.

No matter, though, if you name your cat Dinah, Callie, or, I don't know, Spike, someone's going to call her him and him her. It's easy to get mixed up about feline gender, after all, since cats don't hit you over the head with secondary sex characteristics. No peacock's tail, lion's mane, or three-inch heels. Their appearance is more or less gender-neutral, a neat androgyny, which makes a name like Sasha so apt.

So why do they get called "she" more often than "he"? One friend can't break this habit even with her very own cat, despite the fact that she's the one who gave him the unambiguously male name Barney, and I am convinced Sasha would get called "her" even if I had named him Boy, like Tarzan's son. In the collective unconscious, it seems, cats must embody a feminine principle, and even the most beat-up old tom must endure the ignominy of the feminine pronoun. A *New Yorker* cartoon that shows two dogs watching a cat stroll by tells it all: "What do cats want?" one dog asks the other, in an echo of Freud's famous query about women. Or as the paper boy we had when I was a child once told my mother, "Eeewwhh, cats are for girls!"

Like the macho-man-in-training that he was, the paper boy had a dog. Even the word "dog" suggests the masculine, for a female dog is not a proper dog but a "bitch," whereas a male dog is Dog unadorned. It's the opposite with cats. There's a special word for the males, "tom," and while breeders use "queen" for the females, I've never heard it used conversationally. A female cat is just "cat" (unless, of course, she's "pussy," but let's go no further with that), as if the word itself in some essential way whispered "girl."

For all their testosterone-driven intensity in the real world of dueling toms, "catfights" have come into the language as spats—by implication, petty ones—between women. "Dogfights," by contrast, are white-knuckle tests of courage for World War I flying aces of the male persuasion. Even the Egyptians, great cat lovers that they were, saw a female principle in cats. The cat-headed goddess, Bastet, had the body of a woman.

The identification of cats with the feminine makes me wonder if the ascendancy of the cat today bespeaks a kind of subversive victory for the female, a little-noted chink in the clanky old armor of the patriarchy. After all, we happened to get a cat—a male, to be sure, named Socks in the White House after a long, long string of dogs just when we also got a First Lady with actual power.

Lest we stretch the feminine analogy too far, however, it should be noted that there remain diehards on the other side as well, people who insist on the masculine pronoun—like my grandparents as they named their cat Elmer—no matter the Zeitgeist or the evidence in front of their eyes. Like exiled Russians who still believe the Romanovs will return, they are as stubborn in their use of "he" as those who keep calling Sasha "she."

"He had kittens," a member of this school told me recently, an old woman who despite her confusion dearly loved her cat. "He had kittens, so we had to have him fixed."

*   *   *

It's amazing—or appalling, really, since it speaks of the vast number of abandoned animals there are—that so many kittens find homes the way Sasha did: by soliciting on the street, relying (as it were) on the kindness of strangers. My other two cats are variations on that theme, and most of my cat-owning friends got their cats in much the same way. "Found puppies and pound puppies," as one friend, who has a cat and three dogs, puts it.

It takes a certain amount of chutzpah, a decided lack of timidity, for a cat to reach out and paw an unknown human, jump in her car, and drive away with her, as Sasha did with me. How far these cats have come from the ways of the creature they descend from—the cautious, solitary wildcat, whose idea of prudence is to run away from humans, not toward them. If survival of the fittest is the name of the game, then the cats deemed "fit" in our postmodern world may well be the cute, friendly, self-confident ones—cats with enough sass to approach a stranger and enough charm to be chosen by one. With this assist to natural selection, we humans may well be shaping the evolution of the species, linking the cat's destiny to our own.

Food is the main thing on the mind of a stray, so perhaps it was the meatball that clinched the deal as far as Sasha was concerned. I sometimes wonder whether it was I who picked out Sasha or he who picked out me. The facts seem to suggest the choice was ultimately his, and I merely allowed it to be realized. One of my friends named his cat Circe to memorialize her extraordinary seductive skills—like Sasha, she picked him up at a restaurant—and when you hear enough of these stories you start believing that the Sirens who bewitched Odysseus' crew weren't sorceresses at all, but cats.

Of course, it's flattering to be singled out for attention, even if only by a cat, and perhaps Sasha got me to open that fateful car door for him on that dark Rhode Island night by giving me this particular form of gratification. He made me believe *he* thought I was special—and since I desperately want to believe that I am, in fact, special, corroboration from any quarter is welcome. From this perspective, the experience smacks not of feline guile but of mutual validation. Sasha made me think well of myself by thinking well of me, so I returned the favor by thinking well of him. It's actually not so different from how I choose my friends. Like everyone else, I like people who like me. I like the folks who seek out my company, for this speaks to their good taste and discernment, and these are the friends whose company I in turn seek out.

That little calico stray who lived with me briefly used similar tactics on the electrician who rewired my kitchen. She flirted with him outrageously. She climbed into his big black tool case, which he had opened on my kitchen table, rolled over on her back atop the wire cutters and screwdrivers, and waved her paws in the air adorably, inviting a tummy rub (a familiarity cats will allow to only a trusted few). She followed him about as he worked, weaving silkily around his ankles and gazing up at him with big, soulful eyes.

The poor guy didn't stand a chance. "Are you sure? Are you sure it's all right if I take her?" he asked over and over, as if he couldn't believe I'd let such a specimen go. Then he got on the phone and called his wife, who agreed that it might be kind of nice to have a cat, and off the two of them went. I never did find out what he named her.

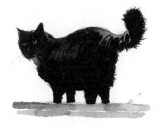

# 4 Approach/Avoidance

Whoever it was who first put forth the theory that cats prefer a solitary life must not have had cats. It's true that the wildcat flies solo, and most of the big cats do, too, with the notable exception of the lion. But among the domestic variety, barn cats tend to cluster in colonies, and so do strays—like the cats of Rome, who live amid the ruins of Caesar's Imperial City and get fed by kindly Romans. The lion in his companionable pride is perhaps a better model for *Felis catus* than the solitary leopard. A much repeated PBS documentary, in fact, points out many behavioral parallels between a group of African lions and a bunch of barn cats living on a farm in rural England.

Of course, it's one thing for a feline family group to welcome new arrivals in the form of newborn kittens and quite another for a house cat to have a companion thrust upon him by human fiat. When I was growing up, my cat Romeo accepted as a matter of course the little siblings our family cat—his mother, Bean—kept producing, ignoring or playing with them as the spirit moved him and smacking them around a little when their roughhousing got out of hand, just like a pasha, as father lions are called, with his cubs. (I quake at guessing whether, like a feline Oedipus, he actually fathered any of the little tykes.)

As an adult, though, I've witnessed some hair-raising scenes when two unrelated cats suddenly meet, either through a human medium or out on their own. Cat-care books are filled with advice for people who want to bring a second cat into the household, a task that's immensely easier if both animals are young and therefore less heedful of the territorial imperative than full-grown cats. While it's obvious that companion cats deeply enjoy one another's company, the hissing and skirmishing and jousting for position that usually precedes their friendship could well give rise to a suspicion that cats just don't like one another very much. Hence, I suppose, the myth of the cat as a loner.

It takes time, shared experience, and the gradual unfolding of trust—a delicate thrust and parry—to get to know another. Just as we humans must come to our own conclusions about a stranger in our own good time, so must a cat. It's woeful to have a relationship forced upon us, no matter how well meaning the perpetrators, which could be why fix-up dates so often fail so miserably—and why resident cats so vehemently protest the arrival of a newcomer.

◆      ◆      ◆

Psychologists have a term they use to describe the dance we do in first getting to know someone, the tentative moves toward him and the backing away, moving forward again as we get to know him better and again taking a step or two backward until we're surer of where we stand. It's called in their jargon "approach/avoidance," and it's a concept I began thinking about when a new cat showed up in the neighborhood one summer a few years ago—a thin, scraggly tomcat, apparently a stray, whose black and white markings were arrayed in a kind of harlequin design.

The sudden appearance of a black and white cat made me wonder if Sasha was some kind of feline art director, orchestrating an assembly of cats whose variations on the theme of black and white would serve to play up his own. At one point he had waltzed in for a meal with a black and white stray named Charcoal at his heels, and now here was another cat, also black and white, hovering in the background. (It was *déjà vu* all over again when Tigger joined the clan some years later and came home one night with another ginger cat—a dead ringer for himself—in tow.)

I never saw any of the preliminaries leading up to Sasha's friendship with Charcoal, so I cannot speak to the approach/avoidance scenario these two must have played out. My guess is that things went fairly smoothly, impelled by an urgent need on both sides—Charcoal's for a home and Sasha's for a cat his own age to play with. His two companions at the time, Mimsy and Jean Arthur, were by then crotchety old things who kept telling him over and over how much they despised his games, which largely consisted of his chasing them madly around the house and trying to wrestle.

So it was with great interest that I began watching the intricate rondelay between Sasha and the harlequin cat. It was a study in approach/avoidance.

I first became aware of this skittish interloper when he took to creeping into my garden during the evenings several summers ago, his mews drawing Sasha and Charcoal to the front door for a look. Whenever I showed my face, though, he immediately vanished into the shrubbery. For a while I thought he was Buddy, one of the neighborhood cats, stopping by on his rounds. But that would have been strange behavior, since Buddy and Sasha had long ago settled the question of whose territory ends where. Gradually I got a better look and saw that this cat was an unknown quantity, a new kid on the block.

After a time Harlequin (as I'll call him for narrative clarity) grew a little bolder. Now I would find him out in the yard, a respectful distance from Sasha and Charcoal but clearly engaged in silent interaction with them designed, it seemed, to test the limits of their tolerance. Charcoal is quite mellow by nature and doesn't much mind being number-two cat in the household—Chester to Sasha's Matt Dillon. He let the stranger get fairly close. But Sasha, as top cat, did not.

If Harlequin invaded what Sasha considered to be his personal space—first fifteen feet, then ten, then six—Sasha charged him like a splendidly antlered buck facing down a challenger who's trying to take over the herd. The charge was fierce but abruptly halted. He would skitter to a stop, his rear quarters fishtailing a little like a semitruck whose driver just slammed on the brakes, right in front of where Harlequin stood. This aggressive posturing succeeded in causing the new cat to bow his head Japanese-style, the feline signal of deference, and back off very, very slowly—too speedy a departure could have provoked a chase—to a site more to Sasha's liking a little bit farther away. There he would sit, and watch and wait some more.

Sometimes Harlequin came by, meowing, late at night, when I was reading in bed with the two cats asleep beside me. Both would instantly awaken, Charcoal giving the tentative, low-pitched growl he usually reserves for the times when the dogs down the hill start barking in unison, and Sasha leaping onto the shelf that's built into the little loft bedroom's half-wall, to look down on the living room and make sure the cater-wauling did not issue from inside the house.

This courtly exchange went on for several weeks, until I began to see that Harlequin had gradually become more of a welcome visitor, and less of a nuisance, to my cats. He was starting to make himself at home on my property, and instead of chasing him away, Sasha now loped right up to him—the speed of the sally was the only hint there was still some aggression at play. Then they would sniff-touch the whiskery spaces beside each other's noses in the universal cat salute, a delicate gesture that always reminds me of society ladies or Frenchmen wanly kissing the air beside each other's cheeks.

This cat was clever, I thought, in the ways of approach/avoidance. He had practiced on my cats what amounted to deconditioning therapy, of the sort that a therapist might use with a phobic. If you're phobic about snakes, for example, your therapist might show you a children's-book picture of one, then a more realistic rendering, then a toy snake, and so on until you're ready to encounter the real thing. In just the same way, Harlequin had imposed his presence on my cats in small, manageable doses. Always courteous, ever deferential, this feline diplomat proved the non-threatening nature of his intentions many times over during all the charging and bowing and backing away that went on between him and Sasha.

It didn't take much longer for Sasha to fully accept him, and by now I would often find all three cats sitting side by side on top of my wood pile in meditative silence, like three black-robed monks sitting Zazen.

Sasha drew the line at letting him in the house, although Harlequin tried. One night I called for the cats to come in, only to find him emerging with the other two from out of the shadows, so close that Sasha was forced to turn several times and charge, lest Harlequin trot right up the fieldstone walkway to the door.

I myself once let Harlequin know that too much familiarity can be unwelcome, not to mention rude. I was weeding and watering the garden one evening with Sasha and Charcoal beside me and Harlequin looking on from his perch atop the woodpile, when after a while my two cats drifted away and vanished up the road. The moment they were out of sight, Harlequin crept into the edge of the garden that's closest to the woodpile and lowered himself into the position that signals "I'm about to take a dump"—right beside the thriving patch of catnip that Sasha and Charcoal so love.

Although I don't usually interfere in my cats' social life, I found myself, in a fit of loyalty, turning the hose on Harlequin. He scampered off before he had a chance to territorially mark the cherished catnip patch with his droppings.

Being spritzed didn't chase the harlequin cat away for good, but something must have, for once summer turned to fall I no longer saw him around the neighborhood. He vanished as mysteriously as he had arrived. But although the cat himself was not with me, his lesson remained. Harlequin had shown me that feline introductions *can* go smoothly if there's plenty of room—spatial, emotional, and temporal—for the approach/avoidance spiral to play out. When there is, integrating a new cat into the household can proceed without a hitch, as I discovered when Charcoal, and later Tigger, joined mine. When it doesn't, the results can be a nightmare, as I found out only too well when I first brought Sasha home.

Awaiting him at the apartment in Brooklyn where I was living at the time were two thirteen-year-old female cats who would become his housemates for the next two years, until the summer that both of them died. Mimsy and Jeannie had been with me since they were kittens, through good times and bad.

They had moved with me three times, from Illinois to Manhattan to Brooklyn, and were about to move again, to Pennsylvania. In short, they deserved a little gratitude and a nice, quiet life. Instead, I brought home a kitten.

*        *        *

I had read somewhere that you should have a friend carry the newcomer in so your cats won't condemn you as the traitor who visited this horror upon them; and this I did. The book also advised leaving the new cat in his carrier for a while as you and your friend drink tea, chat, and pretend not to notice that your resident cats are sniffing around the cage and snootily turning up their noses, as if a spaceship had dropped a particularly loathsome cargo of aliens right in the middle of their living room. This I also did.

But Sasha didn't make it easy on me. He yowled, and he clawed so indignantly at the metal bars of the cat tote that finally my friend was compelled to release him. He burst into the room the way Mighty Mouse would zoom into the scene on his Saturday-morning cartoon show: chest puffed out, hands on hips, and a big goofy grin on his face. And Mimsy and Jean Arthur were never the same from that moment on. No manner of encouragement from me could ever convince them that Sasha was anything less then the hideous beast they knew him to be in their hearts.

At just about six months old he was, in retrospect, exactly the wrong age for them—too old to be seen as a kitten, pesky but inconsequential, and too young to have put away childish things. He was, shall we say, frisky. One friend said that if Sasha should buy a car, the state of Pennsylvania would delete one letter from the license-plate motto it used at the time to make it "You've Got a Fiend in Pennsylvania."

Sasha wanted friends, he wanted playmates, he wanted to

rock and roll—and if you didn't know better you would have thought his rough, exuberant games were expressly designed to deeply alienate two thirteen-year-old females of the lace-doily school of cat behavior. The fact that he was smart, funny, affectionate, and really really cute cut no ice with them at all.

I knew what Jeannie and Mimsy were going through on warm nights when I had to cover up with the winter quilt to protect my toes from Sasha's nocturnal attacks. It was impossible to work at home on any project involving papers—a big disadvantage for someone who makes a living as a writer—without first devising defensive measures to preempt his gleefully plunging into the neatly stacked manuscript and scattering the pages all over the floor. (I turned in articles studded with pinpricks that came not from the removal of misplaced staples but from kitten teeth.) Sasha's headlong leap into Mimsy and Jean Arthur's life couldn't fail to repulse them, in much the same way you may suddenly resent the man you've been dating because he's beginning to steamroller all over your life like a one-man blitzkrieg. Sasha seemed to think taking over the empire was his Manifest Destiny, and, like two dowager princesses, the other cats were not amused.

It didn't help that I was living in a one-bedroom apartment in Brooklyn Heights at the time, with no outdoor space for a rambunctious kitten to let off steam. And I confess that in desperation I called on the services of a cat psychologist.

It was humbling to admit defeat. I had always lived with cats and fancied that I knew them inside out. I certainly had no trouble introducing Mimsy and Jeannie to each other back when Mimsy was a kitten of about Sasha's age and Jean Arthur was a littler kitten. For a few days, maybe a week, the two would offer perfunctory little hisses every time they passed each other in the house where I was then living in Illinois. After that Mimsy took over. She would fussily care for Jean Arthur, washing her as methodically as a mama cat when the two curled up together for their naps. Outdoors, she proved to be something of a natural hunter and would bring the big grasshoppers she caught over to the more inept Jean Arthur in order to teach the littler cat the ropes.

But the misery Sasha was causing my two loyal old friends called for drastic measures, and so the cat shrink came to call. For a mere $150, I think it was, this very nice man in a suit—an animal behaviorist with a Ph.D. after his name—came right to our home for a consultation, the way Columbo visits the crime scene to scope out the suspects. Sasha, who always enjoys company, cavorted on his giant, carpet-covered scratching post while Dr. X was visiting, but Mimsy and Jeannie retreated to the bedroom like children snubbing an unliked relative.

Basically, the doctor said, the trick is to mimic as far as possible the deconditioning spiral that would occur naturally if the cats had met in the wild and got to know one another over time—the kind of thing I later witnessed between Sasha and the harlequin cat. Aping this process is no easy matter in an apartment or even a house, because cats, who are highly territorial, feel threatened when an unknown Other enters their domain. Meeting a stranger in the neutral no-man's-land of the woods or on adjoining suburban lawns is one thing; but having him plop down in your living room and make himself at home is a serious affront.

Dr. X, however, offered one concrete suggestion. He recommended separating the warring animals in two rooms divided by a door, and using that door as a medium for a nonthreatening exchange. Saw off an inch or so from the bottom of the door and dangle a string or ribbon underneath it to encourage the cats on either side to play, he said. They will see only paws on the other side of the barrier and associate them with the pleasures of the game.

You keep sawing down the underside of the door a little bit at a time so that the adversaries gradually see more of one another's bodies. These fuller but still partial views will remain non-threatening, the doctor explained, because cats have trouble with field-and-ground perception. It seems only if she sees another animal in its entirety does a cat register that she is in the presence of the Other, the enemy. As in the Indian fable of the blind men with the elephant, a solitary leg, tail, or ear remains an abstraction.

As satisfying as Dr. X's remedy was in theory, it proved less than efficacious in practice. I am somewhat mechanically inept and found it hard to envision how I was going to keep taking my bedroom door off its hinges, sawing it down, and then putting it back up again. And where would I keep the cats while this activity was going on? The door was metal, anyhow, and although I suppose I could have used a hacksaw on it, an inner voice told me the building's management might not approve.

I did, however, adapt the doctor's advice in my own way. I kept the combatants in separate rooms whenever I was away from the apartment (a tactic that demanded multiple food dishes and litter pans, but at least left Mimsy and Jeannie unmolested in their own home). And I experimented with the string-and-door game.

First I dangled under the door a length of grosgrain ribbon long enough to give purchase to the cats on either side. Then I moved up to dangles through a door opened gradually wider and wider, but barricaded so that Sasha couldn't hurtle through the opening into Mimsy and Jeannie's bunker, as he kept trying to do.

Sasha thought the string game was a lot of fun. And Mimsy batted gamely at the twitching green ribbon now and then, though she couldn't be induced to really throw herself into the sport. As for Jean Arthur, I'm sorry to report that she steadfastly refused to participate in any way other than giving me the evil eye whenever I tried to sweet-talk her into taking a swipe at the ribbon. No matter what Dr. X had predicted, Jeannie seemed to know that the little white-tipped paw making feisty passes under or alongside the door was nothing less than the Claw of the Beast.

Jean Arthur was immovable. This, after all, was the cat who had thrown a hissy-fit when she came face to face with the life-size photo of a calico in my cat calendar one year.

◆   ◆   ◆

Fortunately for all of us, we very soon left Brooklyn behind and set up housekeeping in northeastern Pennsylvania, where I bought a cottage—a real fixer-upper—in a little community just across the Delaware River from New Jersey. It's less than two hours by car to New York, more exurban than rural, but compared with New York City it will do.

Here the cats had a house that gave them a little bit of elbow room, plus three quarters of an acre of their own property to roam and the yards and woods surrounding my neighbors' houses to explore. In this territorial tabula rasa, they settled into something like an armed truce after the overt hostilities of Brooklyn, and I cemented the armistice by decreeing that whenever they weren't outdoors they would occupy separate living spaces.

Sasha, who was more interested in real-world adventures than the two older cats, needed continual access to the front door, so he got the living–dining–kitchen area on the main floor. Mimsy and Jeannie had slept with me nearly every night of their lives, so they got the loft bedroom plus a small room leading up to it that is thankfully separated from the rest of the living space by a door.

This Solomon-like division wasn't cast in stone, so the

three cats ran into one another from time to time both indoors and out—most notably at the food dish, for everybody ate in the kitchen. But tempers had cooled enough so that mostly these encounters produced no hysteria. The cats had become accustomed to one another's presence; the deconditioning spiral had largely played itself out.

Still, whatever their forbearance, it was clear nonetheless that as much as Mimsy and Jean Arthur might tolerate Sasha, they really did not like him. Maybe they never forgave him for disrupting their peaceful lives. Maybe they resented having to compete for my attention with this spirited young rake. Or maybe it was one of those cases where you just can't stand someone on sight, and deeper knowledge of his character, revealed over time, fails to reverse that fateful first impression. Unlike Elizabeth Bennet, who did a 180-degree emotional turnabout in *Pride and Prejudice,* Mimsy and Jean Arthur never found anything at all to admire in the Mr. Darcy that Sasha represented.

The older cats' disdain was a matter of some concern to Sasha. I would go so far as to say that he actually seemed pained at being so thoroughly spurned. He was baffled, too. After all, didn't he try his best to win these two over by continually thinking up games for all of them to enjoy?

The flaw in his reasoning was that the behavior he felt to be play, Mimsy and Jeannie interpreted as aggression. One favorite was Let's play chase, a pretty standard form of entertainment for kittens and young cats—all three of mine get a boot out of it to this day.

Sasha would set off after whichever victim happened to appear whenever he was in the mood for a romp, and when she bolted off in alarm, he unfailingly believed he had finally gained a convert. He skittered along merrily behind her, an expectantly playful gleam in his eye, only to be rebuffed anew—usually by a hiss coupled with a sharp swat on the nose. This is a reproof a cat well understands, because when he's a kitten his mother reprimands him with this very slap.

Mimsy was a gorgeous, haughty, broad-shouldered part Maine Coon, whose thick black and white coat made her look like she could, in fact, have been Sasha's mother. She was big and authoritative enough to dispense with him easily. But Jeannie was a nervous, high-strung little thing who cowered and trembled and yowled and flew off in a panic, generally behaving as if it were Satan himself, and not a young black cat, that was chasing her down.

As for Sasha, he invariably looked demoralized after one of these episodes. Whatever Mimsy and Jeannie were trying to tell him, he just didn't get it, and—as for so many of us when it comes to life's hardest lessons—no amount of repetition was any help at all. He usually found it best at these times to make himself scarce by going outside for a while.

◦    ◦    ◦

Jeannie was undoubtedly a little neurotic, but she made up for it by being exceptionally beautiful. Part silver Persian, she had long, silky gray fur that mixed the mottled stripes of her prosaic parent with the incrementally blended shading—from tips of slate gray to roots of near white—that is the hallmark of the purebred side of her heritage. I've often imagined it was her undeniable beauty that made this little princess an obscure object of desire for Sasha. Or maybe it was simply the adversarial challenge that she posed. At any rate, once we moved to the country Sasha decided that Jeannie, the cat who disliked him the most, was the very cat whose company he most longed for.

On long winter evenings he sat on the couch and gazed up at her as she perched flirtatiously on the shelf that's built into the loft's balcony-style wall, overlooking the living room. Very soon he discovered he could get closer if he jumped on top of a china cupboard that then stood against the living-room wall, beside the door that led up to the bedroom. There he would position himself and stare, as Jean Arthur looked down like Rapunzel in her tower, with no hint of her usual scorn.

Night after night Sasha sat atop the china closet that first winter in Pennsylvania, and after a while I began to suspect that he might be scheming for a way to gain entry to the Forbidden City. Sure enough, his next maneuver was to begin standing upright atop the cupboard, stretching as far as he could on his hind legs and reaching upward with his forepaws toward Jeannie's elusive presence.

This wasn't far enough, of course. Beneath the cathedral ceiling, the wall measures nearly fourteen feet from the floor to the top of the balcony. Simple mathematics tells you that a six-foot china closet topped by a cat outstretched to his full eighteen inches or so still left at least six and a half feet between him and the spot that so obsessed him. Sasha had never even leaped directly from floor to cupboard; he always used the arm of the couch as a launching pad. Surely there was no way he could muster a sheer vertical jump of this magnitude. Jeannie didn't seem to think so as she sat watching his continual machinations with great calm.

One night while I was sitting on the couch watching TV with a companion, I heard Sasha begin to make scratching noises in the area above the china closet. I glanced over my shoulder to note that he looked more frustrated than usual at his inability to scale the wall, and was scrabbling around in an apparent attempt to find a toehold. I was turning back toward my friend when I suddenly caught, out of the corner of my eye, a streak of black motion that looked like the launch of a miniature, fur-bearing space shuttle. This was followed by a great thud.

My companion and I raced upstairs to find, amazingly enough, that Sasha had finally succeeded in achieving his long-held goal. This supreme athletic effort had depleted him, though. He sat where he had landed, plunk in the middle of the bedroom rug, looking as dazed and exhausted as an Olympic pole vaulter who has just set a new record and is badly in need of Gatorade.

As Mimsy and Jeannie stood on the bed in wide-eyed astonishment, like cartoon elephants startled by a mouse, my friend and I brought Sasha back downstairs. He didn't seem hurt, so we gave him cat treats as a reward for his derring-do and then got out the tape measure.

From the top of the cupboard, Sasha had skyrocketed seven feet, one inch—or about the height of Kareem Abdul Jabbar—over the balcony and into the bedroom. I wonder if I can get him into the *Guinness Book of World Records*.

❖     ❖     ❖

I fully believe that Sasha's extraordinary act represented much more than a kittenish prank, or a winter's evening diversion. This great, improbable leap upward into the world of the other cats was born of profound frustration, perhaps even despair. It was Sasha's way of expressing how deep was his need for companions of his own kind. The lack of such communion in a setting where it would seem to be available in such abundance—a mere whisker's breadth away—must have been hard for him to bear.

Sasha just plain needed a friend. And he found one in Charcoal.

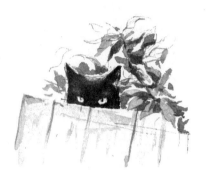

# 5  One Hungry Cat

Where Charcoal came from I don't really know. He just kind of showed up one day perhaps a year after our move to the country, a specter made manifest by the intensity of Sasha's wish for him to be there.

He came home with Sasha, who trotted in the door that autumn day as if there was nothing at all unusual about showing up for dinner with a strange black cat in tow. Charcoal scuttled along behind him to the food dish but kept one eye trained on me, ready to turn tail and run if things should turn ugly. It's scary to go where you're unsure of what your reception will be, unless you're very, very friendly—or very, very hungry. As it turned out, Charcoal was both.

He ate and ate. He would clean out his own dish, and wait politely until the other cats were finished so he could nose around in theirs for any dabs of cat food they might have left. Once in a while he stuck his head in Sasha's dish while Sasha was still eating. Perhaps because it was he who had invited Charcoal in, Sasha was tolerant of this breach of manners, at most giving him the kind of look you might give an uncouth dinner guest who was using his fingers instead of a fork on the mashed potatoes.

Lions and the other big cats understand the feast-or-famine mentality. They gorge themselves happily when they've downed some prey and then endure a fast until the next successful hunt, and this was the style that Charcoal brought to the food dish in my house. It took a good long while before he fully believed that the daily miracle of the ever replenished kibbles would not give way to an empty bowl tomorrow.

◆  ◆  ◆

Given their intense reaction to Sasha's arrival, I didn't know what to expect when Mimsy and Jean Arthur found yet another strange cat in their home. To my surprise, they didn't seem to mind. And clearly, Sasha had led the pantherlike newcomer to our door; they already seemed best of pals. Considering this a tacit okay from all three of the incumbents, I started feeding Charcoal, and he's pretty much been a fixture around here ever since.

One reason he fit in so well was his personality, which was definitely not Type A. Polite, affectionate, and easygoing, Charcoal was what you might call a plain-vanilla, no-frills feline—Shakespeare's "harmless necessary cat." Handsome without being beautiful, neither overly bright nor overly stupid, he wasn't much bother to have around except for getting underfoot whenever anyone went into the kitchen. He was a couple of years old, probably more, at this point, so he must once have lived around people. For unless a cat is lovingly handled and well socialized as a kitten, he grows up wary and skittish, the independent cat of myth, like my grandparents' Elmer, the one we called "wild," or the barn cats at the farm stand down the road.

Charcoal made himself pleasantly unobtrusive. He accepted without question that as an outsider, he was low cat on the totem pole, and in his dealings with the other three cats, he was deferential to a fault. He would quickly jump off any chair that one or another of them wanted to sit in, for example, locating an alternative spot that he always seemed to find just as satisfactory as his original choice. He followed Sasha around with obvious devotion, and was always in the mood for whatever adventures the other cat might cook up. If Sasha went out, Charcoal did, too. When Sasha came in, so did he.

And he left Mimsy and Jeannie alone.

With me and any other humans who might be around he was almost painfully ingratiating, gratefully accepting whatever attention came his way and cheerfully putting up with indignities the other cats would never tolerate, such as being decked out in ribbons and dolls' clothes and getting toted around by one friend's young daughter (just like Romeo when I was a little girl). It was this child who gave Charcoal his name.

By this time, the Berlin Wall separating upstairs cats and downstairs cats was crumbling, and finally I decreed that the door between their enclaves would be opened. Any concerns I had about taking this radical step quickly vanished, for time had worked in my favor—and Charcoal's presence helped. As it turned out, this good-natured cat affected the balance of power in auspicious ways.

First of all, with Charcoal around, Sasha now had a buddy of his own, which cured him of constantly supplicating Mimsy and Jean Arthur with his offers—inevitably refused—of rough-and-tumble friendship. This was a relief to us all. Then, too, the cat constellation was more symmetrical with Charcoal in attendance. Instead of aligning themselves two against one, the cats now divided down the middle in two dual partnerships: a pair of older females and a pair of younger males—"the girls" and "the boys," as I took to calling them.

I've just been reading the zoologist Cynthia Moss's book on East African wildlife, *Portraits in the Wild,* and her report makes me think that male-male and female-female alliances like the ones my own cats formed might be the natural prefer-ence of cats. I may have inadvertently stumbled onto something that suited my domestic brood the day I let Charcoal in the door. Moss says that among lions, cheetahs, and leopards alike, same-sex chums are commonly seen but male-female friends are not—except, of course, during mating. This tendency is particularly distinct among cheetahs, who in terms of sociabil-ity fall somewhere between lions gathering in prides and leop-ards living alone.

When cheetah cubs are old enough to live independently, Moss says, a young female will frequently opt to remain with her mother. The two form a family unit, living and hunting together. But males are excluded from the feminine alliance, so male cubs often set off in the company of a brother, or else join forces with another young male they meet along the way who finds himself in the same situation. The Darwinian odds favor the females. The cheetah mother is more skillful a hunter than even a full-grown cub, and she shares food with her daughter as the young cat hones her own predatory skills. But by bonding in pairs and hunting in tandem, the young males boost their own chances of bagging game.

Of course, it's always hard to generalize about cats, much less draw any conclusions from the example of their wild brethren. The big cats themselves continually confound the scientists who study them by eliciting such a wide range of behaviors in their social lives and every other aspect of existence; you're seldom on solid ground making simplistic statements about them. How much more difficult the whole thing becomes among domestic cats, selected and bred by humans over several thousand years for physical and personality traits that we might consider appealing.

In the realm of male-female relationships, for example, I can't help but recall that Romeo and Bean, the cats of my childhood, lived happily together for many, many years. Unlike a cheetah mother, Bean saw no need to kick her son out of the house; and unlike a cheetah cub, Romeo didn't befriend the other male cats in the vicinity—not even Pinky, his half brother from an earlier litter, who lived around the corner with the Millers.

And friends who have long kept Siamese cats tell me this breed prefers living as male-female couples, behaving like loving spouses even when both of them are neutered. Their cats, Duchess and Cocoa, are the very picture of devotion, keeping up a stream of conversation, as Siamese do, as they follow each other around the house, as if to constantly monitor each other's thoughts and opinions. The more timid Duchess frets and fusses terribly whenever bold, blue-eyed Cocoa goes outdoors without her.

⁂        ⁂        ⁂

Although feline life in my newly integrated household proceeded more calmly now than it once had, there were still some rough patches to get through. The main area of wrangling centered on me. As the only human in permanent residence, I was the one that all four cats turned to for strokes, literal and otherwise. And try as I might to attend evenhandedly to everyone, I had only so much time and attention to go around.

The rivalry was strongest between Jeannie and Sasha, for by now, like many a spurned suitor before him, Sasha had come to dislike the object of his affection. Just as neurotics sabotage themselves by behaving in precisely the way that's guaranteed to bring about what they most dread, so Jean Arthur's continued antipathy had turned Sasha into exactly the enemy she feared he would be.

I could understand Sasha's dislike; Jeannie *was* annoying. She still hissed and spat whenever she met up with him, and her histrionics were so out of proportion to the stimulus that even my sympathy was starting to wear thin. Also, she was an attention hog, a cuddler who wanted to sit on my lap or be carried at my shoulder, like an infant being burped, every waking moment of the day. Since Mimsy had never been a lap cat, her companion's obsession never was an issue in all the years the three of us lived together. But Sasha seemed to take it as a personal affront.

Sometimes he tried to force Jean Arthur from my lap by charging at her the way I later saw him charge at the harlequin cat, either so he himself could come up for a cuddle or—at least so it seemed to me—just for spite. At other times he would acknowledge the fact that Jeannie got there first, while making it plain he was far from pleased. His two favored ways of conveying this message were to march ostentatiously to the front door and demand to go outside (which served to evict Jean Arthur from my lap, momentarily anyway, while I got up to let him out); or to sit across the room from us, on top of the TV, and glower at the distasteful spectacle before him.

Charcoal remained on the sidelines as this battle of wills went on. He must have known that with three other cats vying for my attention, he didn't have much of a chance. Charcoal was the cat in the middle, the silent onlooker, and I didn't pay him too much mind. I fed him and let him in the house, but I told myself that despite evidence to the contrary he was not really "my" cat. Who needed four? Three cats were more than enough to handle, and sometimes too much. When anyone asked how many cats I had, I always said three and a half. Charcoal was the half.

Of course, this was partly his own doing. Charcoal didn't stick around full time, but would show up, hang out with Sasha for a few days or a week, and then disappear for a while. I see in retrospect that this pattern was just like roaming Romeo's; it signified nothing more than "unneutered male." At the time, though, I nourished the hope that Charcoal might have a "real" home elsewhere, and was only stopping by in a series of prolonged social calls.

But in the months following Charcoal's first appearance at my door, three events occurred to change the picture irrevocably. First of all, Mimsy and Jean Arthur both died, leaving the planet the summer they were both fifteen in pretty much the same order in which they had entered it. Mimsy went first. She suddenly grew quite thin, and before I had a chance to get her to the vet's she left the house one morning and never returned. I scoured the neighborhood looking for her to no avail, and I assume she must have gone away to die.

Jeannie, meanwhile, had been a sickly little thing all her life, spending more time than any cat should at the vet's. She deteriorated fast after Mimsy's disappearance, and finally I felt I had no choice but to have her euthanized, the first (and, I hope, the last) time I ever had to make that wrenching decision. Maybe it was my obvious distress, or maybe it's something they always do for bereaved owners; but the vet and his assistant kindly sent me a sympathy card after this awful event.

The next trauma was Charcoal's. Following a fall and winter during which he was at home with me and Sasha more often than he was away, Charcoal suddenly showed up one fine spring day with a broken back left leg. Animals have an amazing tolerance for pain, and Charcoal was stoic about his injury. He seemed just as cheerful—and just as hungry—as usual, despite the fact that he was hobbling around with his leg hanging weirdly off the ground at a crooked, unnatural angle. When I took him to the vet's, X-rays showed that shotgun pellets had shattered his thigh bone. I never found out who was responsible, and whether Charcoal was shot intentionally or by accident.

Dr. Dubensky wasn't sure if he could save the cat, but in the end he performed remarkably delicate surgery, and Charcoal is still with us to vouch for the vet's skill. He barely even limps. In fact, the only visible consequence of his injury is that the claws on both of Charcoal's back legs no longer retract, a trait he shares with cheetahs and with dogs.

I decided to have Charcoal neutered during his three-week stay at the veterinary hospital to curtail his wandering (and ensure that he wouldn't add to the population of unwanted kittens) and thus, finally, assumed responsibility for this wayward animal. However it had happened, Charcoal was officially mine.

❖   ❖   ❖

We now went through another period of adjustment. After Jeannie and Mimsy's deaths, Sasha had settled in to what he must have considered the best of all possible worlds. As only a semi-permanent resident, Charcoal provided companionship but no real competition, so Sasha got to experience the glory of being an "only" cat. In no time at all he grew quite jealous of our exclusivity. So when Charcoal returned from the hospital with a metal pin (later removed) in his leg and full privileges of membership in the household, Sasha found it necessary to lay down the law. Charcoal must be taught that he, Sasha, had prior claims on me. And most of the tussling took place at bedtime.

Sasha decreed that Charcoal was not to sleep with us—he was welcome to curl up on the bedroom rug or on the quilt atop the cedar chest, but he got chased away if he tried approaching the bed. It seemed to me that this tiff went beyond the territorial, that there was a whiff of something approaching sexual jealousy in it. Said one of my friends at the time, "Sasha doesn't think he's the baby, he thinks he's the boyfriend," and it's a thought that a couple of boyfriends have seconded since. My next-door neighbor, Isabelle, once had a similar experience when a boxer dog by the name of Caesar grew so possessive that he would let no one else come near her. One afternoon she was lying on the couch nursing a headache with the ever vigilant Caesar by her side. He successfully prevented Isabelle's husband, Bill, from getting close enough to deliver two aspirins.

Perhaps because Charcoal was such an obliging sort, this period of wrangling did not last long. I'd like to think my own strategy of non-intervention helped smooth the way. My belief was that Sasha and Charcoal should settle their questions of dominance and status themselves; I guess I had learned an important lesson from all my useless meddling in Sasha's political battles with Mimsy and Jean Arthur. I tried to take my cue from the cats. Since Sasha had been here first, I treated him with the same respect that Charcoal did. When I fed them, Sasha got the first scoop. When I gave them cat treats, Sasha got the first one (and the last). When I greeted the two cats, indoors or out, I petted Sasha first, then Charcoal. In the arena of the bedroom, I took Sasha's side and agreed that Charcoal should stay off the bed.

It seemed to work out just fine. One morning around this time I woke up to find Sasha purring loudly on my chest and

Charcoal lying at my side—for his persistence wore Sasha down, and after a while he was allowed to sleep on the bed too. I began petting both cats, and the overflow of affection this brought on sent Sasha right over to Charcoal. The two cats exchanged nuzzling head bumps just the way that lions do in the elaborate greeting ceremony they perform with members of the pride upon waking from a nap. Charcoal then started grooming Sasha, methodically washing the other cat's face and ears with his rough pink tongue. Mother cats lick their kittens this way, kittens groom each other, and African lions, according to Cynthia Moss, wash one another's faces too.

Being licked by its mother's tongue is the first tactile contact a newborn kitten has with the world, its first encounter with the universe of other beings, and grooming remains a sensuously gratifying experience for cats of every size. Some believe the reason cats so love to be petted is that the human touch approximates the rough licking they once received from their mothers. Based on the blissful faces of Sasha and Charcoal that morning, it's not hard to agree.

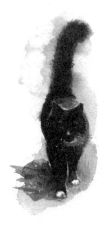

# 6 Sasha's Tail

The single thing that everyone who meets Sasha notices first is the way that he carries his tail. He typically walks around with this magnificently long, luxuriantly feathered appendage held proudly aloft like a flag, a posture that augments the sense of grandeur with which he presents himself.

This tail is indeed a remarkable organ. Functionally, it serves him as a kind of rudder. Repositioning itself as the animal jumps or falls, the clever tail is largely responsible for a cat's fabled ability to land on his feet.

Aesthetically, it's a thing of beauty, two inches in diameter and wispy as milkweed.

And expressively, it's an eloquent tool. Sasha speaks volumes with his tail. He flicks it in what can only be read as impa-

tience when annoyed, whips it about wickedly when he's mad.
When he concentrates on something, the tail concentrates too.
It stretches out rigid behind him as he stalks prey, twitches
thoughtfully as he stops, ears pricked, to listen for some elusive
sound.

Outdoors, he raises it in a visual "Hello!" as soon as he enters a magic circle of his own imagining that extends, like a
spotlight beamed on a lone performer, three to five feet around
wherever I happen to be standing. "Here I am!" the tail says, in
a throwback to the signal of recognition kittens give whenever
they see their mothers—a mannerism that reminds me of the
colorful flags Sistine Chapel tour guides carry so their groups
can easily spot them amid the swirl of other tourists. (The analogy is not so far-fetched: Mother leopards with cubs trailing
behind them in the tall grass of the African plains loop their
tails up and forward over their backs; since the underside of a
leopard's tail is almost pure white, it acts like the beam of a
lightship guiding sailors through a grassy sea.)

There is a protocol to the raising and lowering of the tail.
This is a conscious greeting, not a random one, for Sasha typically lifts his tail only if we have made eye contact or he is walking directly toward me. And only within a certain range. Outside the circle that Sasha envisions around me, he keeps his tail
down; when he crosses the perimeter, it rises as surely as the
tide. Like the moon, I affect its ebb and flow, for I have the
power to expand the circumference of the circle with my voice.
When Sasha hears me speak, especially if I say his name, he
immediately lifts his tail in response, even if he's outside the
usual confines of the circle. Not *too* far outside of it, though. If
he is, say, fifty or a hundred feet up the path in front of my
neighbors' houses, he bounds toward me with tail stretched
parallel to the ground, and only raises it when he is ten or fifteen feet away.

When Sasha is investigating something—examining the

crevice in a stone wall that a chipmunk has just ducked into, for example—it will not let him be. I speak, and up the tail goes, but it's down again in an instant. I say another word and it rises again—and just as promptly falls. The tail has a mind of its own. It's like a very polite person who feels he must return your greeting even as you interrupt him in the middle of some important task.

◈    ◈    ◈

But the tail has another tale to tell. It's also a marker of status and authority, and to fully understand Sasha's character, status must be taken into account. For Sasha is top cat. He is the boss cat in the household, the big enchilada, the cat-in-chief. He is the alpha cat, to borrow the term biologists use to denote a dominant individual in, say, a wolf pack, and as such he is daily preoccupied with questions of status and submission.

You don't have to be a particularly astute observer to notice this cat's air of authority. It hangs about him like an aura—charisma, feline-style. I myself fell into its thrall that dark October night when Sasha introduced himself outside a Rhode Island restaurant and convinced me, against all rational judgment, to take him home. Tigger saw it, too. For the first couple of weeks after he came to live with us, the kitten would literally quake in his boots whenever he caught sight of Sasha, even though the top cat was not at all aggressive toward him. At dinnertime Tigger ducked into the narrow space between the pie safe and the kitchen workstation, and poked his head out just a little bit to sneak a peek at Sasha as he ate. Nothing could induce him to come get his own food until the top cat had licked his chops and gone back outside.

Sasha has star quality. You see it in his face, in his posture, in the self-confident way he moves through the world. Sasha doesn't walk, he struts. This is partly due to biomechanics—his back legs are slightly knock-kneed, giving him a swaggering, gunslinger's gait—but it's just as much a matter of attitude. You see it in his self-assured dealings with other cats, with humans—even with dogs. And you see it in his tail.

There's something so prideful—so bold—in the way Sasha carries his tail that it seems to shout self-satisfaction and high spirits. Tail erect, he's Jupiter brandishing his trident, a drum major leading a parade, or Charlie Chaplin twirling his cane. My friend Beth, newly returned from a wolf-watching trek in northern Minnesota, found a parallel in the upright-tail stance that tells observers (and other wolves) at a glance who is top animal in a wolf pack, and her interpretation gains credence in light of the fact that Sasha raises his tail not only when he greets me, but also when he approaches Charcoal and Tigger (who don't follow suit in approaching him or each other, although they do raise their tails for me). The kittenish explanation might do for a cat saying hello to a person, but it doesn't hold water for a top cat greeting an underling.

It's hard to read this tail when it comes to relations with the other two cats. Sometimes Sasha saunters up to them with tail held high in a friendly greeting; the next thing to happen will be head bumps, the feline equivalent of shaking hands. But sometimes he approaches with tail high and body language that seems to bristle, then jumps on top of them and wrestles them to the ground in a show of dominance. Let's hope Charcoal and Tigger are better at decoding the tail's meaning in regard to themselves than I am.

*     *     *

In the end, it was probably Sasha's top-cat manner more than any other single quality that got him into so much trouble with Mimsy and Jean Arthur. They were his elders, they were fully grown, they were residents of long standing in a home he joined after being rescued from a panhandler's life at the restaurant. Why didn't he show his gratitude the way Charcoal later did, by lying low and being as accommodating as possible?

Instead he seemed to feel he had a right to rule the roost, and Jeannie and Mimsy resorted to nose swats in an attempt to teach him his place. The only trouble was, he knew his place, and it was on top. Mimsy and Jean Arthur never managed to convince Sasha that he was anything less than the certain privileged Someone he knew himself to be. He set himself up as top cat, and finally they had to accede.

My friend Barbara, who raises Huskies, has been watching a similar situation unfold in her home ever since the birth of a dog named Hooper. From the start it was clear that this pup, one of two males in a litter of five, considered himself the top dog. He elbowed his way to the top of the puppy heap with an attitude of ascendance so pronounced that a group of us looking at puppy pictures before we met the dogs in person all commented on it. His siblings went on to other homes, but Hooper stayed with Barbara, growing into an enormous dog who cheerfully bosses around his two canine companions—his mother, Blaze, and grandmother, Ranger—just as Sasha did in my house with Jeannie and Mims.

My friend offers a theory to explain why Hooper is so presumptuous. It seems Blaze labored long and hard to deliver the sibling born just before him; then Hooper surprised everyone—including his mother—by popping out with no further ado, like Venus springing full-blown from the head of Zeus. With no birth trauma to teach him that life means hard knocks, postulates Barbara, Hooper has every reason to believe the world is his oyster.

The Hooper Theory, though unprovable, is worth thinking about simply because it *is* an explanation, or at least an attempt at one. Otherwise, you're left pondering a stew of imponderables: the elusive mix of genetic and/or environmental factors that might (or might not) explain why one cat or dog, and not another, behaves as if the rest of the world should acknowledge his preeminence. You might just as well ask why Bill Clinton and Jimmy Carter grew up to be presidents of the United States, while Roger Clinton and Billy Carter did not. It's the nature/nurture puzzle, in all its perplexity, revisited in animal form.

In Sasha's case, being male no doubt has something to do with it, for male cats tend to be more status-conscious than the females—an outgrowth, it seems, of the need to protect territory or risk losing turf to more macho males. Indeed, questions of status and dominance never seemed high on the agenda for Mimsy and Jean Arthur, who maintained, as far as I could see, a pretty equitable balance of power throughout the fifteen years they lived together. Each was ascendant in her own way—Mimsy so splendidly self-assured that you might have considered her the top cat, and Jeannie so persistently demanding that she often managed to wrest more than her fair share of attention from me. They were like the eccentric aunts in *Arsenic and Old Lace,* sometimes querulous but mostly affectionate.

But when Sasha joined the household, he began defining relationships in hierarchical terms. Deborah Tannen points out in *You Just Don't Understand,* her best-seller on male and female conversational styles, that men talk to establish status and independence, while women talk to establish rapport. This is a generalization, to be sure, but it more or less held true in the "conversations" among my male and female cats.

Charcoal showed up as if on cue to assume the number-two slot in the pecking order Sasha had devised—you can't be a top cat without a second banana to bear witness—relieving Mimsy and Jean Arthur of that burden. And this placid cat, he who was regularly chased off the bed in the early days of his life with

Sasha and me, still validates Sasha's assertions of power. In Sasha's mind, it appears, Charcoal's role is crucial. His very existence as perennial second fiddle is living proof of Sasha's entitlement to be number one. And so Sasha must continually stage-manage reminders that he himself is top cat and Charcoal is not. The result is regular rumbles, of a sort I never witnessed when I had female cats alone.

For example, on a recent occasion Charcoal was fast asleep atop my grandmother's knitted afghan, which is draped over one end of the couch in my sunny workroom at the house's lowest level. Then Sasha came in from outdoors and, with absolutely no provocation, lit into him. He jumped on top of Charcoal and the two began rolling around in a heap of kicking claws. They tumbled to the floor and rolled around some more, growling and yowling under the coffee table—then separated as suddenly as they had come together. Sasha now took the superior position, as he almost always does, standing above Charcoal with one lethal paw frozen in front of him, ears back, and a "Make my day" expression on his face. Charcoal lay on his side with his stomach exposed—a posture of submission—and raised his fists defensively.

At this point I picked Sasha up and whisked him over to the desk, where I held him on my lap and stroked him in an attempt to break up the brawl. No way. He struggled out of my arms and went right back to Charcoal. The two set at it again, tumbled around for a while across the carpet, and then tore up the spiral staircase to the main floor of the house—Charcoal in the forefront and Sasha in pursuit.

I heard more thudding and thumping, then silence. Sasha now strolled casually back down the stairs, tail swaying as serenely as a palm tree on a tropical beach, and headed over to the very afghan where Charcoal had so recently been sleeping. Curling up for his own nap, the victor baldly laid claim to the territory of the vanquished.

Later, when I went upstairs to make myself some tea, I found Charcoal snuggled up with my Raggedy Ann doll on a ladderback chair in the dining room. Neither cat appeared the least bit upset by the altercation or any the worse for wear, despite the little tufts of black fur that I found scattered about in their wake. Maybe they both find it comforting to be reminded, from time to time, of exactly who they are.

❖   ❖   ❖

Whatever the role of testosterone, and the impact of territoriality, these can't be the sole determining factors in the making of a top cat, or Charcoal and Tigger would be just as presumptive as Sasha. Moreover, I've seen the same noblesse oblige in females, including Beanhead, who remained the authority figure, cat-wise, in the household I grew up in despite the presence of a big tough tom named Romeo.

My friend Sherrie's tricolor Persian, Misty, who briefly stopped by my place the day Sherrie got her, is a top cat, too. It happened to be dinnertime, and despite being in an unfamiliar house surrounded by unfamiliar people and unfamiliar cats, Misty pranced over to the lineup of food bowls in the kitchen with tail held high and nose in the air. Just a few months old and weighing in at three pounds tops, she was a real princess in training. My own cats—and I had four of them at the time—were so nonplussed at her display of hauteur that they simply stared at this exceedingly fluffy apparition in mutual astonishment.

If age and gender are not barriers to adopting the attitude of an alpha cat, as Misty showed, then incumbency isn't, either, as Sasha proved in asserting himself over cats who preceded him into my home. Nor is size the determinant. Mimsy was bigger than Sasha, who at ten pounds falls within the high-average range for domestic cats. So are Charcoal and Tigger, but they bow nonetheless to his authority.

I'm tempted to conclude that a top cat simply is born that way, for I can see no "nurture" issues to explain why two cats as disparate as the purebred Misty, who was raised in a Persian cattery, and the no-breed Sasha—who was living out of a restaurant dumpster when I found him—would assume the same regal manner. However, I can think of one exception that makes me believe some top cats can rise to the rank and need not assume it from birth.

This would be my mother's cat Ralph, a shy, broad-nosed, brownish tiger with enormous double paws who looks as if he stepped out of a nineteenth-century American folk-art painting. For the first seven years of his life Ralph played sidekick to a very large tiger cat named Carleton, to whom he was devoted and to whom he deferred. But now Carleton has died, and Ralph finds himself unexpectedly thrust into the alpha position with my mother's new cat, an impish young Tonkinese (they're a cross between Siamese and Burmese) named Randall. Just as Carleton laid down the rules for Ralph, so Ralph is assuming this task with Randy. And he seems to like it. My mother reports that Ralph is a much more self-confident cat these days, and a friendlier one, too. With no intermediary shouldering him aside, he is more expressive and affectionate, much more of a "people" cat than he ever was before.

Ralph may not be to the manner born, the way that Sasha is. He seems a bit unsure of himself in the top-cat role, the way Gerald Ford always seemed slightly astounded that through a bizarre twist of fate he was President of the United States. Nevertheless, reports my mother, Ralph has quite suddenly adopted the tail-aloft salute, a posture she never noticed him using when Carleton was alive.

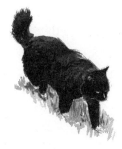

# 7 Comings and Goings

It's a Sunday morning in early October, a warm but cloudy Indian Summer day enlivened only by the shrill reds and yellows of the first-turning trees. Sasha wants to go out. Having wolfed down the cat food du jour I scooped out for his breakfast, he is eager to plunge into the new day and whatever adventures it may bring. He marches to the front door, just as he does each and every morning at around this time, sits down smartly on his haunches, and stares at the doorknob. His long white whiskers arc forward, doorward, but that is the only sign the cat gives of what is on his mind. He does not meow or scratch or otherwise betray impatience, for he knows I can be counted upon to open the door, this hinged barrier between him and the world, and deliver him to the outdoors. His morning leavetaking is an ingrained part of our daily routine.

An hour has gone by, and now I hear the familiar rattle signaling that Sasha has returned to leap acrobatically onto the top quadrant of the old, wood-framed screen door. He wants to come in. I laugh out loud, as I always do when I see him this way. Spreadeagled on the screen, hanging there by his claws and sheer weight of will, he is at once imperious and slapstick. From this vantage point he is just about my height, and for a moment our eyes meet through the scrim of the screen. I ease the door open, and Sasha releases his grip. He lands on the walkway with a soft, graceful thump and strolls inside.

First he rubs his cheek proprietarily against the old farm table that stands just inside the door, renewing his scent on this gateway to home. Then he veers over to Charcoal, who is stretched out on the living room's braided rug. Much more the homebody than Sasha is, my number-two cat has remained inside all morning.

The two exchange head bumps with so much enthusiasm you'd think they had been parted for days, not an hour or so.

"I'm back!" "Welcome home!" is the wordless exchange.

Sasha then goes into the kitchen, where I next hear him crunching on dry cat food. At times like these he never eats much of it, and I've come to believe he heads for the kibbles not out of hunger but to reassure himself that the always filled bowl is still there, still full—that all is in order and the house is just as he left it.

Satisfied, he ambles back out into the living room and jumps on the coffee table, craning his neck forward toward where I am sitting on the couch and reading the Sunday paper. I rub him about the head with short, brisk strokes that must feel to Sasha much the way Charcoal's nuzzlings did.

By now he's been indoors for all of five minutes. Apparently that's enough. He jumps off the coffee table and heads once again to the front door. He wants to go out.

* * *

A couple of hours have passed and this out-in scenario has repeated itself twice more. One excursion outdoors was prompted by the vacuum cleaner. Like many cats, Sasha seems to believe this loud, ungainly instrument was invented expressly to vex him, and whenever I get out the Electrolux he flees. Now I am downstairs in my workroom with the door leading onto the deck wide open to let in the day, which has begun to turn sunny. Sasha comes in.

His eyes are as round as an owl's and his body language speaks contained excitement, as if he is a cat who has seen amazing things. "If only I could tell you!" his expression seems to say, and he trots over to the desk where I am working for the requisite greeting and petting.

Then he heads for the louvered doors that open into a large storage area tucked into otherwise unusable space between the main floor and the downstairs of the house, and scratches impatiently at them. Here is a set of doors before which he must make his intentions clear—unlike the front door, where he manages, in silence, to draw me whenever he wants out.

I get up to oblige him now, opening one of the louvered doors so that Sasha can slip into the storeroom. For reasons unknown, he finds this dusty place, jammed with cardboard boxes and stored furniture, fascinating and worth repeated exploration.

I return to my work, and after a while I get up again to see if Sasha is still in the storeroom. He is not. He must have gone back out.

A half hour later I myself go outside to greet a visitor, only to see Sasha burst out of the bushes at the far end of the gravel path that runs between my house and several of my neighbors'. He races toward us, face expectant and tail raised high.

Has his feline radar signaled that his human has opted to enter his domain, the great outdoors? Or is he guided by some inner clock that leads him home at appointed intervals, the fact that my friend and I are outside to meet him being just a happy coincidence?

After rubbing joyously around my ankles and those of my friend, Sasha trots resolutely to the front door and stands there, staring meaningfully at the doorknob.

Surprise! He wants to go in.

◆    ◆    ◆

What is it about cats and doors? Surely everyone who has a cat—one that is not housebound, that is—has noticed their door compulsion. It's pretty hard to miss. If a cat is in, he wants to go out. If he's out, he wants to come in. Or so it seems to us humans, slavish keepers of the gate for these restless, whimsical beasts.

The repetitious exercise of the door takes on the weight of metaphor, for the door is the bridge between the two worlds in which a cat finds himself: the domestic interior, that place of warmth and comfort where his loving humans dwell; and the wide, wild spaces of the bigger world, the world of nature that is his birthright as a cat. The relentless passage between these two realms, as represented by the opening and closing of the door, hints of an underlying unease, as if the cat must constantly strive to reconcile some primal dislocation. In the home but not of it, he seeks the outdoors. In the wild but with longings for the hearth, he wearies of his travels and feels an urgency to return, the perennially prodigal son.

Lately I've been observing Sasha outdoors in an attempt to see whether he is a noticeably different creature outside than he is in—more wild, somehow, or otherwise transformed from his domestic self. There can be no totally objective study, however, because when I can see him, he can see me, and my presence undoubtedly influences his behavior. In fact, Sasha gives every appearance of being extremely happy to see me whenever I go outside into his turf, and he seems to have a sixth sense about it. Often enough he'll suddenly materialize from wherever he might have been to join me as I work in the garden or sit reading on the deck.

If I take a walk along the neighborhood's narrow gravel roads, he trots along behind me. I once would have thought it odd to hear of someone going for a walk with a cat. But when we moved to the country and he was allowed outdoors, Sasha showed me that cats enjoy walking as much as dogs do. Often Charcoal joins us, too, although he is not as bold as Sasha and becomes increasingly uneasy the farther we get from the house. He hangs back and meows unhappily, then sprints nervously forward to catch up with us, and then hangs back again, describing an edgy, eccentric orbit. (His anxiety stems, I believe, from the trauma of being shot a few years back, when Charcoal was still a stray. Clearly, in this cat's experience, home and its immediate environs are safe, the bigger world is not.)

Now I have a third cat, and Tigger, too, trots along behind me like a small red shadow when I walk. Sometimes, if the cats happen to catch sight of me at the same time, all three of them gambol along in my wake, turning a simple excursion into a merry parade.

But there's many a day that Sasha goes outdoors in the morning and disappears for hours, whether I am outside or in. I don't know exactly where he goes or what he does on these lengthy sojourns, though I know that hunting for mice and birds and chipmunks—basically, anything that's smaller than him and moves—is a part of it. I also know that he frequently makes visits to some of the neighbors, 'for one or another of them will tell me that the cat stopped by to see them while they were raking leaves, hanging laundry, sitting in the sun, weeding the garden. Sasha is a very sociable cat and has his favorites among the folks around here—notably Cory, a robust retired gentleman, born in Holland, who lives three houses away from us. His wife, Elfriede, tells me Cory sometimes saves scraps from dinner to give Sasha the next day. The cat has become a neighborhood character, as much a part of the tapestry of life here as I am myself.

Not long ago I discovered a surprising addition to Sasha's outdoor repertoire. I went outside on an unseasonably warm autumn day and found him curled up for a cat nap in a clump of sun-drenched weeds in front of the woodpile, ten yards or so from the front door. I've seen him sitting, at rest, on the deck railing, lounging atop the woodpile, lost in thought on the stone wall across from the house—but never before had I actually seen him fast asleep outside.

The reason this nap so surprised me is that I have noted one characteristic in Sasha the outdoor cat that is substantially different from his indoor attitude: a kind of hypervigilance, as if all his senses were instantly tuned to a higher frequency the moment he walks out the door.

When he first leaves the house in the morning, for example, he moves smartly onto the front walkway or veers off into the garden right beside it, then stops. He looks about keenly and sniffs at the air, as if getting the measure of the day. His ears stand at attention, twitching slightly as he listens for sounds that I do not hear. Vague rustlings in the leaves? Birdsong? The music of the spheres?

His eyes narrow, his pupils black slashes in an amber field, and while I realize this is a physiological accommodation to the sunlight, it makes him look shrewd and feral, totally unlike his indoor self. Outdoors, he gives the impression of being master-ful—more powerful, somehow, than the companion creature who lives with me in my house.

The transformation, if there is one, is this: my cat becomes in appearance what he is in fact. An animal.

*     *     *

It has crossed my mind more than once that Sasha knows our property and the surrounding landscape much more intimately than I myself do, or ever can. He is closer to it, literally—by dint of his size—and in the gifts of sensory perception that are his. From where Sasha stands, the gaillardia that is still bravely blooming in October is more than just another clump of garden flowers. It is a substantial bush, a verdant presence. It rises like a canopy over his head, a living parasol, where to me it barely brushes the knee.

As I bend down to nip off the deadheads, Sasha rubs against the plant's thick, nubby stems, gingerly mouths some of the lower leaves, raises his head to sniff and examine the under-sides of the daisylike blossoms. I look down at their cheerful yellow faces and at his face beneath them. It's all a matter of scale, but if God is in the details, then Sasha is closer to Him than I am.

The cat leaves the gaillardia and me behind. He makes his way through the garden, onto the path, and up the embank-ment across the way, there to stretch full-length against a young tree in what looks like a vertical version of a yogi's morn-ing asana. (He often performs the classic horizontal position as well—the rump-up, torso-down, arms-outstretched greeting of the sun—and one wonders if the founders of yoga devised this sinuous, vertebra-by-vertebra stretch after observing it in cats.)

I suddenly feel a touch of envy, for there is something so right in the way my cat approaches his world, a Zen-like manner of moving through the landscape and with it, that I become bumptious and awkward in comparison. Sasha is at home here; I am not—or not quite. He fits. I am too big to navigate the same trails that he can travel so lightly.

However much he may be a part of it, though, the connection to the sensory world must be reestablished with every footfall, every breath. Hypervigilance. Sasha heeds each sound, sometimes with alarm, always with attention. He catches every shift of the wind. He pauses frequently to sniff the ground, noting every scent for what it might tell him about the passage of other animals—cats, dogs, the wild things that are prey or competitors or foes.

This world is intensely, electrically alive, it crackles with an energy we human are too preoccupied to heed. Every tree, every rock, every clump of weeds has information to convey. Every object speaks.

In one graceful movement, Sasha descends the embankment and jumps from the stone wall that fronts it to the gravel roadway below. The sun has soaked this patch of road, cooking it to a temperature and consistency that pleases the cat. He throws himself down upon it and begins to wriggle, rubbing first one side of his body and then the other full-length in the warm dust. Back and forth and back again he goes, flexing and unflexing his supple spine as he flips from side to side until he has given himself a gravelly rubdown—a full back and body massage.

He rises, rapturous, in a cloud of dust and twigs and shreds of autumn leaves. They cling about his long black fur in a dusky penumbra, like the force field that surrounds Pigpen in the *Peanuts* comic strip. It seems peculiar that so fastidious an animal would intentionally make himself dirty by rolling around in the dust, but cats seem to find nothing paradoxical in it. All three of mine enjoy a bracing road rub whenever they can manage it, although the other two don't seem quite as transported by the experience as Sasha.

The cat walks over to me but seems distracted now, as if his thoughts are elsewhere. He gives me a perfunctory rub about the ankles, taking no notice of the fact that he's getting me dirty in the process, and accepts a scratch about the ears in return. Then he turns tail and heads down the road and into the woods. I know that by the next time I see him, no speck of dust will remain to mar the perfection of his coat.

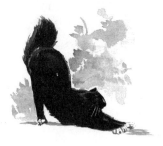

# 8  Sasha's Turf

There are two things to be said about walking with Sasha. The first is that he does not advance in a straight line. The second is that he knows his boundaries.

I discovered the former trait when I first moved to the country and, foolish me, bought a little blue collar and leash in the hope of supervising Sasha outdoors, to keep him from running away or getting lost. But Sasha found the leash mortifying—an insult of the first order—and I can't say I blame him. Walking on a leash does not suit a cat's natural style. A cat is just not built to trot alongside you in a straight line at a measured gait. Nor is he meant to be restrained.

Leashed, Sasha would zigzag down the road in a manic

stop and start, brought up short—in a motion that looked suspiciously like whiplash—by the limits of his tether whenever I failed to keep up with him. After that he would sit, and refuse to budge. He was stonewalling me.

I've always marveled at how expressive a cat's face can be given that there's not much there to work with. A cat's face is small, after all, and covered in fur. Cats have no access to smiles, tears, eyebrows, laugh or frown lines as aids in conveying emotion.

Yet despite the apparent lack of raw materials, they manage to express a wide and subtle range of feelings that punctuate the Buddha-like demeanor that seems to be standard issue for a cat. One of these expressions is disgust. When deeply offended to the point of disgust, a cat scrunches up his face and flattens his nostrils in what looks like an aristocratic sneer, the way a member of the English royal family might should he find a mouse doing the dead man's float in a soup tureen.

This was the expression I saw on Sasha's face when he was in bondage to the leash. The experiment did not last long; the leash made us both unhappy.

Unleashed, Sasha has the freedom to decide whether to walk with me or not, and it speaks, I think, to the quality of our relationship that he usually chooses my company. He's not interested in a linear experience, however. He apparently believes the travel itself, the process, is what counts, not the end result. He darts ahead of me or drops behind, veers off to the right or to the left of the path, throws himself down in the road for a dust bath, climbs or scratches at the occasional tree, and otherwise investigates whatever it is that might capture his attention along the way. In between he weaves about my ankles, and if I'm not paying sufficient attention to his whereabouts, I bump into him.

Whatever his meanderings, though, he does not lose sight

of me or depart too far from the line of march. He reminds me of the way Miles Davis weaves his horn over, under, and around a melody but never loses connection with the theme. It's no wonder the jazz musicians of the bebop school called one another "cool cats."

As for boundaries, I gradually became aware of how important they are to Sasha's sense of himself once we began taking walks together. It was through our walks that he informed me of the limits of his territory, the invisible borderlines that make one yard in this neighborhood home turf and the next one suspect terrain.

By my rough accounting, the area Sasha has staked out for himself embraces twelve to fifteen acres that include eight or ten yards of varying sizes, three or four wooded lots that the new zoning regulations deem too small to build on, and an acre or two of rough, woodsy hillside that runs behind my house and stretches out north and south from there, meeting up on the northern end with the road leading into the national park that borders our small development. This slice of territory is no less real, its borders no less distinct, for being unmapped anywhere but in Sasha's head.

Not surprisingly, his own house and yard stand at the epicenter of Sasha's terrain. Home is . . . well, home, no less for Sasha than for me. But the house is not the geographic center. That's because the rutted byway we call the Lower Road, where three or four large, noisy dogs live, forms something of a natural boundary right behind us. Stretched out east-west at the foot of the hill upon which my house is built, the Lower Road forms the bottom line (assuming a bird's-eye view) of the elongated rectangle that is Sasha's domain. Our house and yard sit forward, just left of center, on this imaginary line.

The short leg of the rectangle on the east end rests a hundred and fifty yards or so from Silver Lake Road, the county road off which our development is situated, and runs parallel to it. From a cat's perspective, Silver Lake Road is inhospitable: noisy, confusing, and above all exposed—there's no cover here should one get chased by a predator, such as a dog or a car. It's a good place to avoid, and I can report with great relief that all three of my cats do.

The top (or front) line of the rectangle cuts through various yards and lots within the development. There is no obvious reason why Sasha would have set this particular boundary line where he did—no Grand Canyon, geologic or man-made, to separate home turf from terra incognita. Maybe he used distance from our house as a guideline. His working hypothesis might have been, say, that five house lots (or whatever the equivalent is in cat terms) from his own front door is appropriate wandering space, but six is too far to risk.

The final, western leg of the rectangle is formed by the gravel road that leads down the hill past a few houses and into the park and its series of waterfalls, walkways, and picnic tables. All told, this is a kingly estate for a small cat, a varied landscape filled with diversions and rich in hunting potential.

❖　　❖　　❖

Sasha is a confident, self-satisfied cat within the limits of this territory, and he works hard to keep it that way. Like a rancher riding the perimeter of his property to see that the fences are in good repair, he constantly patrols his turf to make sure everything is in order. Particular signposts have taken on meaning: favorite trees and rocks, the woodpile, sections of the old stone walls that crisscross the neighborhood in an irregular latticework. These he apparently sees as markers upon which he must reinforce the fact of his existence here by freshening his scent.

The skinny young locust by the woodpile, for example.

Sasha often subjects this tree to a vigorous bout of scratching, for not only does it feel good to shred the papery bark, it also deposits scent by means of glands in the paw pads.

The rose of Sharon trees I just planted are too puny to scratch, so these he rubs, marking by means of the scent glands in his cheeks, first one side and then the other, just the way he marks the furniture in the house. A tree unmarked is just a tree, but a tree that's marked is an ally, a sentry informing anyone else who passes (assuming their sense of smell is acute enough to catch a whiff) that Sasha has passed through this property. I imagine it works the other way, too, reassuring Sasha that the familiar slice of landscape he has carved out for himself is still, in fact, his own.

Releasing urine is a more emphatic way to accomplish the same thing, and Sasha frequently marks two particular trees—a birch and an aspen—at the eastern end of our property in this way. He doesn't lift his leg to do it, like a dog. Instead, he raises his tail high and then aims backward and upward, lifting his posterior as high as he can reach as he shuffles his back legs, as if to stand on tiptoe. This is not standard urination, during which a cat splays his back legs, positions his tail horizontally to the ground, and aims downward. Nor is much liquid ejected; only a squirt or two.

Perhaps by aiming high Sasha is hoping to dupe passers-by into believing the cat who did this is a very large cat indeed, someone it would be unwise to challenge in a turf war.

Just how precisely Sasha has set his territorial boundaries began to dawn on me as we took our walks. For example, I often walk to the corner convenience store, which involves following the path in front of the house for an eighth of a mile or so until it veers off down a small hill and spills out into Silver Lake Road. Sasha comes with me, but he invariably stops at the property just past Rossbach's place, at the crest of the hill. From here he can sit on the stone wall and watch me cross the street and disappear into the store. I reemerge, brown bag in hand, and find him waiting in the same spot to walk me home.

Similarly, getting the mail means walking out to where the boxes are set up on Silver Lake Road, a quarter of a mile or so along the development's main drag. Sasha comes with me but stops at Witter's yard or sometimes ventures a tad farther, to Bright's. There he waits till I return, and together we walk back home.

But it didn't strike me how much these limits help Sasha define himself until the day he pushed beyond them. It was our second summer in the country, and a friend and I were walking to the park. We set off up the road with Sasha trotting along at our heels, and made the sharp left across from Witter's to turn down the hill.

Sasha was still with us, but a quarter of the way down he began to behave oddly. It was clear he was determined to follow us as far as we meant to go, but he no longer exuded his usual confidence and control. Instead he seemed nervous, decidedly ill at ease. His face wore a strained expression and he glanced about furtively, like a criminal on the lam. He perched unhappily beside one bush or another along the way, as if unsure about going any farther, and sprinted forward only when my friend and I called out to him to come. He acted, in short, the way Charcoal does when he comes out for a walk—as if danger, not adventure, lurks behind every shrub.

Haltingly, the three of us got all the way down the hill. But when we reached the cutoff to the park we humans took pity on the cat and decided to head back home instead of proceeding with our original plan. So undone was Sasha by this nerve-wracking experience that he actually let me carry him partway up the hill—and being held, much less carried, is something he barely tolerates indoors and rarely tolerates out.

When we reached the top of the hill, Sasha seemed immensely relieved. He wriggled out of my arms and scooted down the road toward the house with all of his usual aplomb, tail erect and self-esteem restored once he had again reached his own territory. You'd never know to look at him now that this cat had just come off a major attack of agoraphobia.

*　　*　　*

Whether Sasha's territory is big or small, typical or atypical for a twentieth-century exurban cat is impossible to say. Male cats, the experts tell us, are more territorial than females and travel farther; unneutered males roam farthest of all. But beyond that broad gender difference, there appears to be no general reckoning of just how much territory a domestic cat demands. The acreage required depends on any number of variables, especially the population density of other cats.

Since they don't demand sheer exclusivity and sometimes divvy up territorial rights in a kind of time-sharing scheme, cats can settle territorial disputes more or less satisfactorily among themselves, even in a cat-heavy locale like the townhouse condominiums where my brother lives and where practically everyone has a cat or two, or three. One bad apple, an unneutered orange male, is notorious for street (actually courtyard) brawls, as Mike's cat, Rusty, can sadly attest. But with that one exception, these Columbus, Ohio, cats have pretty much learned to live in feline harmony without resorting to range wars. Perhaps they adhere to the same principles as the Indians who named a lake in Webster, Massachusetts, Chargagogmanchargagog-chagunabungamaug. Translation: I fish on my side, you fish on your side, nobody fishes in the middle.

Sasha was lucky. Unlike Rusty, he found few other cats inhabiting his new neighborhood when we first moved here and thus had the freedom to set boundaries based on his own personal criteria, whatever they might have been. A couple of neighbors had female cats, but they tended to be stay-at-homes who posed little challenge as Sasha began to establish himself. The only real threat came from Buddy.

Buddy belongs to the Kroeners, who live a few blocks away, on a gravel road that runs parallel to the one in front of my house. He's far enough away so that he and Sasha meet only rarely. But one of those meetings—it may have been the first— was a doozy. It took place shortly after we moved here, at a time when I was still fretful about letting Sasha outdoors by himself (remember the little blue leash?) and would go out looking for him if he hadn't been home in a while. On one such trek, I came upon the cat on the broad front lawn of my friend Doris's log cabin, the backyard of which is more or less catercorner to the Kroeners' property.

Hunkered down in a tense crouch, Sasha was uttering an odd, keening sound from deep in his throat, somewhere between a yowl and a whine but nothing at all like a meow. It sounded like a police siren. It would intensify in pitch, then drop off, then intensify again, as if Sasha were practicing scales. Responding in kind was Buddy, a shy, short-haired, white and gray–striped cat, larger than Sasha, whom I assume had long been unchallenged in his belief that Doris's yard was part of his turf. Now Sasha was contesting the matter.

Buddy too was positioned in a low crouch, about three feet away from Sasha, and the cats were glowering at each other like two snarling samurai on a Japanese scroll. Their ears lay flat against their skulls and their lips curled, as if in distaste but actually in the so-called *flehmen* response, from the German word meaning "lip curl." This strange function—which cats, improbably, share with ungulates—is a kind of sixth sense, integrating taste and smell. What Sasha and Buddy were doing was to trap scent particles on their tongues and send them to specialized Jacobson's organs, which are linked to both aggression and sexuality. It's one more way of gathering data about the world.

Both cats kept up the uncanny keening that so often presages a fight, and I started up the steps leading from the path to Doris's lawn, intent on breaking them up. But suddenly I stopped. Perhaps it was simple curiosity—what would happen next?—or maybe I sensed that my intervention would cause Sasha to lose status in the eyes of a rival. But I also had a feeling that despite their fierce posturing, the two cats were not about to rip each other apart—not yet. For cats, as for humans, aggression is more often ritualized than enacted; the image of JFK facing down Khrushchev during the Cuban Missile Crisis is the same in all its essentials as the scene that was now being played out by Buddy and Sasha. This was no battle, although it could have turned into one. It was an intense communication, a bitter debate stemming from the shock each animal felt in meeting up with the other on territory he considered his own.

The two cats kept up their eerie wailing as first one, then the other moved ever so slightly forward in slow-motion shifts of weight and position. Movement by one caused the other to make a compensatory change, equally slowly, in the opposite direction. Then the second cat would subtly advance and the first one back off in a strange, stately ballet that could have become a wild apache dance in the wink of an eye.

So far it was a standoff, and it began to seem as if the cat with the stronger will would win, as in a game of Chicken.

But after another couple of minutes and at no cue that I could discern, Buddy blinked. I don't know why. Perhaps he couldn't take the tension—perhaps Sasha had successfully psyched him out. With no preamble and no sound, Buddy turned tail and galloped off toward his own house. Sasha ran after him, but just far enough to watch the other cat skitter around the porch and hightail it diagonally across the backyard, homeward bound.

Then Sasha turned around and sauntered over to me, the picture of nonchalance, as if nothing much had happened. But something *had* happened, something significant. Sasha had successfully laid claim to Doris's yard, and I have never seen Buddy set foot in it again.

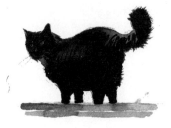

## 9  *Real Dogs Are Big Dogs*

Buddy was the only cat to seriously question Sasha's territorial decisions, but there were others in the neighborhood who had opinions of their own on the subject: dogs.

Sasha doesn't like dogs, and I can't say I blame him. In his experience, the best of them bark, the worst of them chase. There may be a third variety in small, inconsequential (to the feline eye) dogs like poodles and schnauzers, but I'm not convinced Sasha actually sees these as dogs. A real dog, however bothersome or obnoxious he may be to a cat, is a force to contend with. Like a hurricane or a freight train, he can't be ignored. Strategies must be devised to manage him, even if the strategy is avoidance.

But little dogs *can* be ignored, even tolerated. They pose no threat, produce no ripples in the Zen-like Now of a cat's life. The excited yipping of Sandy, the nervous cocker spaniel across the way, evokes no more than a yawn from Sasha, who seems to feel it is simply not worth the effort to respond in any way. And Katy, a good-natured little Toto-like terrier, appeared to be a source of entertainment to my cat during the days she and her mistress lived in our neighborhood.

When Katy and her owner came by on their daily walks, Sasha would examine the dog with what I can only describe as wry curiosity, sniffing and circumnavigating her as if she were an exotic specimen in a zoo as she stood smiling and subservient on her leash. Once in a while he would accompany her on her strolls, picking his way delicately along the stone walls that line the paths as Katy trotted along beside her owner on the gravel below.

In the world of real dogs, the alpha and omega are represented by Sparky and Shawn, big dogs who taxed Sasha's patience and tested his courage during our first years in the country. Sparky, a mischievous young Shepherd-Husky mix who then belonged to my neighbor Tom (and now lives miles away with Tom's ex-wife), humiliated Sasha more than once, a matter of no small import, since cats agree with the Japanese that it is a terrible thing indeed to lose face.

As for Shawn, the German shorthaired pointer who used to live next door, this dog was something of an object of scorn. Sasha figured out pretty early on that this elderly, brown-spotted barker was all bluff. With cloudy eyes and arthritic back legs, Shawn to the end of his days would, on occasion, get up the gumption to chase Sasha the few yards from his property to ours. Sasha's response was to lope a few paces toward home, then turn, with a contemptuous flick of the tail, and face down the dog with studied nonchalance.

"Surely you jest," he seemed to be saying. Whereupon Shawn would duly, if ungraciously, retreat.

It wasn't always so. When we first moved to Pennsylvania, Sasha and Shawn embarked on an extended series of territorial and psychological negotiations regarding status and the rights of free passage. Younger and a little more frisky back then, Shawn at first had the upper hand. Hip-high to a human, he was vastly bigger than Sasha and had the advantage of incumbency to boot. In those days he seriously asserted his standing in the neighborhood by chasing all my cats from time to time—Sasha along with Mimsy and Jean Arthur and, later, Charcoal—having been taught to do so by his owner, Isabelle, and her late husband, Bill.

"Cats would come to the bird feeder and we would tell him, 'Go chase! Go chase!'" Isabelle apologetically explains, in an accent that, after sixty-some years in America, still bears a trace of her native Germany. She never dreamed, apparently, that cats might one day move in right next door.

Whereas Mimsy and Jeannie—who lived most of their lives apartment-bound and dog-free—prudently steered clear of Shawn, the feckless young Sasha set out to get the dog's measure and test his limits. No Neville Chamberlain, he apparently concluded that "peace in our time" was not the answer if it meant you had to skulk fearfully around your own territory on account of a dog.

Sasha was intentionally provocative. He would stroll into Isabelle's yard, knowing full well that this would infuriate Shawn, seemingly in order both to tease the dog and to assess his reactions. He often got chased for his trouble, but Sasha never seemed to mind much. He was gaining insight into how far he could push Shawn and the likely response to various types of incursions. It was all part of a strategic chess match the cat was staging.

It wasn't long before I began to notice that Sasha and Shawn had apparently come to a meeting of the minds and forged a kind of non-intervention treaty that lasted until Shawn's death a couple of years ago, though it was far from ironclad. Basically, the deal went like this: Shawn agreed not to chase Sasha when Sasha was on his own property, but he retained the right to do so whenever Sasha stepped over the line into Isabelle's yard. They constantly tested and reinforced these limits. I frequently saw the two of them eyeing each other from a distance of six feet or so across the invisible boundary they had set, the strain in Shawn's face and posture signaling that he was locked in an intense inner struggle to hold up his part of the bargain. Every fiber of his being yearned to chase; mostly he did not.

On Sasha's end, the fact that he was to consider himself fair game if he strayed over to Isabelle's wasn't much of a deterrent. He pretty much treated her yard as an extension of his own, dog or no dog. At times it seemed as if he was taunting Shawn—daring him to act like a man, so to speak. This must have been unpleasantly humbling for an old geezer who in his salad days was rewarded for chasing cats.

One day I heard an unusual amount of barking next door and went outside to find Sasha perched on Isabelle's porch roof, where he had draped himself languorously atop the gutter like Tenniel's Cheshire Cat lounging in the branches of his tree. Sasha was calmly washing his paws and looking down at the exasperated dog, who barked as though his lungs were too small to contain his rage.

❖   ❖   ❖

The noblesse oblige attitude that marked Sasha's continuing tiffs with Shawn surely would not do for Sparky, who was too young and strong and cocksure to be toyed with. Luckily for my

cats, Sparky did not live in the neighborhood full time. He was
a visitor who showed up with his owner during fishing season
and the odd summer weekend. It was on one of those weekends
that Sasha first met him.

It was a balmy, starlit night, and I was heading over to my
friend Doris's log cabin, two houses away from my place, to sit
on the front porch and have a couple of drinks with some of the
neighbors. Ever since he wrested this territory away from
Buddy, Sasha had considered Doris's place his own. He frequently stopped by to visit, sometimes accepting Doris's invita-
tion to come inside and make himself at home, and he enjoyed
basking in the sun on her white porch railing. (He still does,
though the house has now changed hands; luckily for him, the
new owner enjoys his company, too.) From the porch, when
the sky is clear, you see an almost Alpine vista of the slate blue
Kittatinny Mountains rising in the distance, just over the Delaware River in New Jersey.

And so the cat came with me to the party and soon com-
menced socializing, rubbing up to various neighbors who were
sitting on the porch swing and wicker rockers. He then leaped
onto his accustomed spot on the railing and perched there contentedly for a while.

Until Tom and Sparky showed up.

The dog made a grand entrance, kicking up his heels like
an unbroken colt as he galloped onto the lawn, all unbridled
energy. He stood there grinning, lolled his tongue, looked ea-
gerly about, and yipped.

Cats always seem like powdered-wig aristocrats next to canine *sans-culottes*, and that's how Sasha appeared now as he rose
to stare at Sparky, his eyes wide with alarm, or possibly distaste.
There is a vast existential distance, after all, between cats and
dogs. Cats are all inner-directed elusiveness. Dogs are outer-
directed and straight ahead—what you see is what you get.

Cats are as subtle as Zen masters, dogs as unsubtle as the back-field of the Buffalo Bills. Dogs are extroverts and cats—even the most sociable among them—are introverts; rarely do you see a dog sitting in the meditative stillness that comes so natu-rally to cats. In short, these two animals are on different cosmic wavelengths, and it truly must take a great leap of understand-ing on one side or the other for them to become friends.

Sasha took only a moment to assess the situation before jumping off the railing and disappearing into the crawlspace beneath the porch, where Doris was convinced a skunk made its home despite her best efforts to block the entry by filling in the spaces with rocks. Clearly she had not succeeded, for if Sasha could find his way in, so could a skunk.

Sparky wasn't fooled. Either he had caught a glimpse of Sasha or else he detected his presence by smell. It didn't matter which. For the remainder of the evening he dedicated himself to flushing the cat out of his bunker. He continually sniffed about the underside of the porch, barking and yipping and pawing the ground excitedly. Fortunately, Doris had spaced the stones tightly enough so he couldn't get in. And thank good-ness the resident skunk, if there was one, was not at home at the time.

At one point Sparky gave up and sat down to take a breather on the fragrant, freshly mowed lawn, paws crossed daintily in front of him. Sasha took the opportunity to poke his head out of his hiding place, whereupon Sparky spotted him immediately. Yipping wildly, he began a manic, stiff-legged ga-votte, like a coyote doing a dance to the moon. Sasha was forced to retreat yet again until Tom finished his beer and loaded Sparky into the pickup for the ride down to his cabin.

Fond as I am of Sparky, I couldn't help but feel for Sasha, whose dejection seemed visible in a somehow diminished pos-ture and a skittish, low-tailed gait as he accompanied me back home. How painfully distressing it must have been, and what a blow to his pride, to be cornered in that way by a dog. In front of all his friends, too.

◆   ◆   ◆

Things went from bad to worse the next day, when Tom and Sparky dropped by my house to visit. As it happened, both Sasha and Charcoal were indoors enjoying a midday siesta at the time—only to find, upon being awakened by the knock on the door, the nightmarish visage of their least favorite dog grinning at them from behind the screen.

Never in my years of living with cats have I seen a scene like the one that then unfolded. Apparently believing they were about to be set upon in their own home, the two cats, in the grip of an overpowering fright, set upon each other. The fur was flying quite literally as these normally fast friends snarled and growled and trounced each other, tumbling madly in a savage embrace across the living room and dining room, and then tumbling some more down the spiral staircase that connects the main floor of the house with my workroom downstairs.

When I was a child, my parents drummed it into me never to interfere in a catfight—it's too easy get hurt. But in this instance I knew I had to forget caution and pry my cats apart, because they showed absolutely no sign of easing up of their own accord. Using a broom to separate them, I quickly tossed a thick towel over Charcoal and snatched him away from Sasha's reach. The more mellow of the two cats, Charcoal was the one getting the stuffing knocked out of him.

I carried him upstairs and locked him away in the bathroom, where I set down water and food bowls (Charcoal always feels better when he sees that there's food to be had) and left the towel on the floor for him to nap on. Then I went back downstairs for Sasha.

With Charcoal removed from view he was somewhat more composed, but the hair on his back and neck was still erect and he continued to utter the occasional low growl. I soothed him as much as I could by petting him. I crooned to him—"There, there," and similar monosyllables—in my silkiest voice. Then I carried him upstairs, closed and locked the front door (need I say that upon the outbreak of hostilities Tom had prudently whisked Sparky away?), and put on Mozart, nice and low.

Sasha lay on top of the TV and fell into a deep sleep. It took him fully an hour to recover himself. For Charcoal's part, he looked totally bewildered by what had happened and seemed relieved to hole up in the bathroom until the dust had settled.

❖　　❖　　❖

Although this was certainly an extreme example, there is an aggressive side to Sasha's personality that I find perplexing and sometimes a cause for concern. Clearly it was he who had started the fight with Charcoal and he who retained the upper hand throughout. So the next time I was at the vet's, I surreptitiously picked up one of the pamphlets arranged on a rack for us pet owners to take home. (It's embarrassing to admit, but I didn't want Dr. Dubensky to know I had such qualms about one of his model patients.) Titled *Aggressive Behavior Between Cats*, this little brochure put out by a cat-food company sheds some light on the event.

"When two cats in the household who have gotten along well together suddenly become aggressive toward each other," the pamphlet said, "the problem is generally fear-induced aggression. Neither of the cats seeks the other out, but if they run into each other, both will act startled and attack. Usually this problem begins 'by mistake' or 'by accident' "—e.g., by the unexpected appearance of a Sparky to trigger the terror response.

The booklet went on to say that if the trauma is severe enough, the two cats may be hostile toward each other from then on. Luckily for me, Sasha and Charcoal are not the sort to hold a grudge, and after they had calmed down sufficiently to allow Charcoal's release from the bathroom, they acted as if nothing had ever ruffled the harmony of their relationship.

As for Sparky—well, he got his comeuppance in a big way, though it took nearly a year for this act of feline vindication to occur.

On a late afternoon the following April I was in the middle of a phone call when I heard a suspicious barking outside. Oh no, I thought, that is not Shawn, whose bark I know well. Given that trout season had just begun, the time Tom was most likely to show up, could I be hearing Sparky, returned to tear my cats apart limb from limb?

I quickly put down the phone and opened the door to discover that it was indeed Sparky, merrily chasing both my cats in a west-east direction along the path in front of the house. The trio momentarily raced out of sight in a cloud of dust, like the cartoon Road-Runner evading Wile E. Coyote. But an instant later I watched in amazement as this same parade sped by again—in reverse order.

Now it was Sparky ripping along at the head of the line. He was traveling east to west, ears back and tail between his legs, heading as fast as he could for the hillside that is a brambly shortcut down to the cabin where Tom was staying.

Half a beat later Sasha and Charcoal came into view, running beside each other in mirror image, faster than I have ever seen them run. Ears aerodynamically pasted against their skulls, they looked like Goya's demon cats in his famous anti-war etching *The Sleep of Reason Produces Nightmares*. Sparky was no fool—I'd run, too.

Sparky hightailed it down the hill and the two cats

screeched to a stop, turned, and metaphorically rubbed their hands together over a job well done. Then they marched back home and catapulted in the door.

Charcoal now crumpled in exhaustion. He lay panting on the rug looking slightly shocked, as if he had trouble believing he had done what he had done. But Sasha was all keyed up—adrenaline, I suppose. He strutted about the living room for a good long while, gloating and rubbing excitedly around my ankles as if he wanted me to share in his triumph.

I don't know what psychological turnabout took place in that split second the three animals were out of my view, but whatever it was turned victim into aggressor and gave my cats the mental edge. It must be true that matter follows mind—that we are what we believe ourselves to be, and if we present ourselves that way, others will believe it, too. Sparky surely did.

If I needed any further proof that you don't have to be big to be tough, I got it when Sue, the owner of the local deli, told me her cat, Sylvester, had actually treed a bear. A swaggering gray and white cat who's built like a linebacker, Sylvester is known to be fearless. And this was a young, inexperienced bear, it is true. Nevertheless, pound for pound, claw for claw, and fang for fang, the bear could have had Sylvester for lunch. That he didn't speaks partially to luck, but mostly, I think, to the spell one can cast with Attitude.

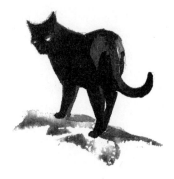

# 10 The Predator at Play

Charcoal chases his tail. It's almost embarrassing to admit this, just as it might be to confess that you still sleep with your Teddy bear or suck your thumb or otherwise hold on to some immature, if comforting, habit you should have outgrown long ago. There's something totally incongruous—anachronistic, almost—in the sight of a muscular, seventeen-pound black cat, who is perfectly capable of savaging assorted small rodents and birds, merrily attacking his own tail the way a kitten would.

Not that Charcoal seems embarrassed. He goes after this beguiling object with great verve, tumbling all over himself and rolling undecorously around on his back in his efforts to nail it, once and for all. Does he have no sense that the temptingly twitching tail is part of his own body? Or does he know that the tail is intrinsic to himself, inalienably his to investigate and enjoy, like an infant playing with its toes?

I've often said that my cats don't play. An assortment of balls, plain and belled; mice, of rubber, plastic, metal, and suede; and indescribable puffy objects made of cloth or yarn lie heaped in a basket, untouched. Perhaps my cats are jaded, beyond such prosaic amusements. More to the point, they are indoor-outdoor cats with plenty of opportunity to discharge in the real world whatever pent-up energy it is that sends their housebound cousins into manic, bop-till-you-drop bursts of activity on a regular basis.

But actually, my cats do play, and I'm reminded of that fact every winter. Winter is an indoor season, and although the cats do pad around over the crusty layer of frozen snow on a daily basis, they stay indoors much longer during this season than they did in November or will in March.

They sit contemplatively with paws tucked underneath themselves, looking like furry philosophers (a posture a friend of mine calls Pawtucket, after the Rhode Island city of that name). They pull up to the wood stove as if it's a kitty TV to watch the fire's hypnotic movements through the glass doors. They find the warmest spots in the house to doze. The living-room windowsill, which is right above a heating duct. A chair in the dining room that stands in front of another heater. The bed, whenever the electric blanket is turned on.

And when they begin to get bored with the sedentary life, they play.

❖   ❖   ❖

There's something enthralling about watching cats at play. You can't take your eyes off them, and you start to understand why actors prefer not to do scenes with animals. They're natural attention-getters, natural clowns, totally unself-conscious and riveting in their single-mindedness.

Cat-owning friends once gave me cat toys for Sasha and Charcoal, little minimalist mice handmade out of buttery suede by some New Age cottage industry. A short strip of rawhide forms the tail, but otherwise these mice have no distinguishing features—no eyes or whiskers or bells, like the toys you buy in the supermarket. They're not cute, and have no pretensions to being lifelike. They're just soft little balls with a string attached.

The cats will ignore them, I thought; these mice will end up in the basket unused, like all the others.

Wrong. For whatever reason, both cats took to these toys immediately—even Sasha, who is hard to please in such matters and no longer chases Christmas ribbon the way he once did when I wrap my packages every year.

The cat attack was swift and merciless. So merciless that both little mice soon disappeared—vanquished into some hidden corner, presumably, or wedged under a low-slung piece of furniture, never to be recovered in this century or until I move, whichever comes first.

The proper way to attack a toy mouse, it seems, is the same way you attack a real one. You pounce on the thing, then throw it in the air, catch it, and hurl yourself over on your side. Grip the mouse with your front paws as if your life depended on it and bobble it in the air from time to time, all the while furiously kicking at it with your powerful back legs. Toss it up again, and when the mouse comes in for a landing lunge, pounce, and bat it madly across the bedroom floor like a hockey puck.

Cognitive dissonance: When played out with a ball of suede as the object of attack, this scene is as funny to watch as a Marx Brothers movie featuring Groucho at his most obstreperous. (My late, lamented cat Melville looked like Groucho at his most manic as he tore around the house with his favorite plaything—the cork from a wine bottle—clamped in his teeth like a cigar.) But the real moves on which this play is based aren't funny at all. This spirited frolic is a rehearsal of the deadly art of predation, and it's something else altogether to watch a real cat-and-mouse pursuit, *Death in the Afternoon* in miniature.

When Sasha, who is a superb hunter, is on the attack, he can become a mad, wild-eyed thing, tossing the prey animal into the air, pouncing on it, then batting it around repeatedly—*toss, pounce, bat, toss, pounce, bat*—until it's too damaged, worn out, disoriented, or disheartened for fight or flight. Scientists who have studied cats tell us this tossing and pouncing and batting is not the sadistic game it appears to be to human eyes. Rather, prudence dictates that a cat must neutralize the threat posed by a rodent's sharp teeth and claws, a bird's talons and beak. To do so requires tiring out, beating up, or otherwise incapacitating the creature so that it can't fight back or run away. It's frightful to watch. I've heard it said that some of these prey animals die of heart attacks, or fright, and I'm not surprised.

What makes it so funny out of context, I suppose, is the very thing that makes it so terrifying in context. Don't humorists play on our personal and social terrors, our dirty little secrets, to make us laugh? The joke becomes funny when we find that we've been let off the hook, allowed to discharge the anxiety it provokes in a cathartic belly laugh. What's dark or tragic or discomfiting in one setting becomes hilarious in another. (Think of the famous B. Kliban cartoon showing a self-satisfied fat striped cat playing the guitar. "Love to eat them mousies, mousie's what I love to eat," the cat sings. "Bite they little heads off, nibble on they tiny feet.")

Watching a cat at play, we forget, momentarily, that what we are seeing is a shrewd predator turning his instincts to an inappropriate object—a bundle of suede or a dangling ribbon—instead of a flesh-and-blood prey animal. The seriousness of the intent is defused by the incongruity of the setting, and we are swept into an alternate universe where the natural order, the drama of life and death, has been turned on its ear.

"Get that mousie," I found myself telling my cats when the

little suede mice were still to be found, so caught up was I in the intensity of their play. "Kill! Get the mouse! Kill!"

*       *       *

Many cat games, if not most, evoke the hunting response. The same friends who gave my cats their beloved suede mice also supplied them with the Cat Dancer, a contraption consisting of a long, supple, curved piece of wire onto which a collection of rolled, cigarette-shaped pieces of thick brown paper are strung. When the cat owner holds this implement by the little wooden handle, the paper end pirouettes bewitchingly just above the cat's reach, tempting him to stalk, chase, and pounce—to the amusement of both cat and human.

Some animals, such as wild dogs, hunt by outrunning their prey. Classified as "coursers," they are nature's marathoners. But cats are stalkers—sprinters, if you will.

Upon spotting prey they lower themselves into a crouch, every muscle atwitch, and watch intently, creeping closer and closer until they're near enough to pounce. Speed combines with the element of surprise as an explosive burst of energy sends them from their hiding place to down the unsuspecting victim.

Such are the tactics that Charcoal uses on the Cat Dancer. Muscles aquiver, ears and whiskers angled forward in intense concentration, he fixes his gaze on the loopy, erratic motion of the paper lozenges—a movement he appears not to connect with me or, indeed, with the wire, as if Charlie McCarthy could walk and talk without Edgar Bergen.

When it's time to go in for the kill, he propels himself forward to grab at the thing. Sometimes he catches it and drags it to the floor, there to claw and gnaw and generally thrash the bejesus out of it. Sometimes it arcs away from him. No matter. He gets a big kick out of the game either way.

Even the habit that some cats have of racing about the

house at a particular time of day is linked to predation, biologists say. If these born-to-boogie hunters don't get to go outdoors and hunt, that pent-up instinctual energy has got to go somewhere. Late afternoon or early evening is the usual time for such jaunts, which figures, since cats by nature are nocturnal beasts. The onset of night is the witching hour.

My cat Mimsy habitually took a crazed but restorative late-afternoon sprint. You could have set your watch by her. The five o'clock express, I used to call it, as Mimsy careened along the long, polished hallways of the first apartment we had in New York. Ears back and paws thundering, negotiating hairpin turns with a great clatter of claws against hardwood floor, the primeval cat was making the best of urban confinement.

◆　　◆　　◆

As entertaining as it is to watch shadow predation unfold in the living room or thunder down the hallway, it's quite another thing to witness the actual event in the world outside your door. It can be a very unsettling experience—sometimes a horrifying one—to watch your pampered pet turn lethal and nab a bird or a mouse. At the same time, I often find myself paradoxically caught up in admiration—a kind of subversive thrill—at the power, grace, and skill this act of hunting entails.

Take the time I saw Sasha and Charcoal hunt in tandem, an act of partnership that is common enough in the big cats but one that I had never seen before—though I have since been told it's not unknown—among the domestic kind.

I was working in the front garden with the cats beside me, when—in unison and faster than my coarse perceptions could register—they suddenly heard, sensed, smelled, or saw something I did not in the tall, thick cedar hedge opposite Isabelle's house next door.

The two cats snapped to attention, instantaneously transformed into finely tuned predatory machines. Both pairs of yellow eyes fixed on a spot in the bushes, both sets of ears pricked upward and angled forward, taut with concentration as they strained toward that spot. In an instant the cats were gone, first Sasha, then Charcoal, launched, almost, like feline cannonballs in a cat circus.

The next thing I heard was a thrashing sound, and then I watched as the cats dragged a bluejay out of the shrubbery. Apparently caught off guard, the big blue bird lay flat on his back, like a patient on the operating table, and beat his wings at the ground in useless protest against the disciplined power of the two black cats.

The cats looked up momentarily with alien, killer eyes— they could have been two lions downing a gazelle on the Serengeti Plains, so far had they traveled inwardly from the quotidian landscape—and the stunned bird made a break for freedom. He dove back into the bushes. The cats dove in behind him. I heard more thrashing, then silence.

Later that day a nine-year-old friend and I came upon the jay's mangled carcass several yards from the site of the attack. We buried it in the backyard, setting down a rock and a couple of blue feathers to mark the grave.

Chilling? Yes, but gripping, too, not least for what it tells me about what I don't know about my cats. How can the lovable creature I live with—this refined and civilized Dr. Jekyll— turn into a Hyde-like beast at the simple provocation of seeing a jay? And where does "my" cat go when this metamorphosis occurs? "My" Sasha is a fluffy, amiable creature with big amber eyes and slightly comic facial markings. He looks as if he should lounge around on a silken cushion all day, not run about killing things.

But when Sasha hunts, he moves beyond the domestic circle, like Kipling's Cat That Walked by Himself. He becomes something wild, primal—Other—a being more ancient and shrewder than man. He reminds me in this way that I do not fully know him, for how can I know the Paleolithic longings of a cat? Nor do I "own" him, for he is not ownable. He is entirely self-possessed.

*       *       *

Yesterday, as dusk was turning to night, I went out to put a bag of trash in the garbage can at the side of the driveway when I heard a familiar quiet rustling, like the rubbing together of corduroy pant legs. This is the noise my cats make as they move about, soft but not soundless, on their rounds. It seemed to be coming from the same bushes, opposite Isabelle's house, where the jay attack had once been staged.

"Sasha!" I called, for he was the only one of my cats outdoors at the time. "Is that you?"

Sasha emerged from the far end of the hedges like a figure in a dream and began walking toward me. His gait was stately and vaguely splay-footed, like that of a pregnant woman, for the chipmunk he was carrying in his mouth threw off his center of gravity.

"What have you got?" I asked, although I could see quite clearly what it was. "Let me see," I said, moving toward him.

But Sasha didn't want me to see. He veered off and crossed into another neighbor's fenced yard, where I could not follow. Never did he alter his ceremonial pace. Never did he lose his expression of preoccupied solemnity, like that of a priest on the way to the altar.

It was a deeply mysterious moment, and I felt for one numinous instant that a barrier had softened between Sasha's world and my own, offering the barest glimpse at something I could recognize but did not understand.

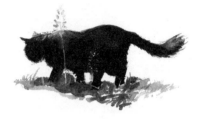

# 11  The Skull in the Garden

One afternoon, digging around in the garden, I came across a curious artifact. Buried just beneath the surface of the soft, rich earth under the azalea was a tiny, bleached, beaked skull that bore, albeit in miniature, the same hollow eye sockets, the same poignant sweep of bone—and the same emotional charge—as the lusterless steer skulls of Georgia O'Keeffe. This memento mori had once been part of a bird, a small one. Perhaps a specialist could have told me what kind. Chickadee? Cardinal? Finch? I did not know, but I carefully lifted the sad little object out of the soil, reflecting as I did on both the abstract, calceous beauty of the thing as it now existed and the act of violence that had made it what it was. This skull once belonged to a living, breathing, singing, flying creature—one who had met a sorry end at the paws of my cats.

Such reminders that for all their cuddly charm cats are predators, first and foremost, have been delivered to my doorstep on a regular basis ever since I moved to the country. As soon as I let him outside, and with a rapidity that astounded me, Sasha turned into the scourge of the neighborhood—Attila the Cat—if you happened to be a bird or small rodent.

How did he even know how to hunt, given that he had lived in an apartment with no outdoor privileges for the better part of a year? Or, to be more precise, how was he able to translate the instincts cats are born with—the predatory moves they show us when they play—into real-world success? How, in short, did he know how to kill? The books say this skill must be taught, cat to cat, so it's possible Sasha's mother trained him when he was a wee thing, well before he came to live with me. On the other hand, it seemed equally possible to me that Sasha was simply a natural, his instincts piqued and talents sharpened by an environment teeming with little creatures that skittered provocatively away at his approach, seducing him to chase.

That, plus practice, practice, practice.

Perhaps in a remote environment—the wilds of Wyoming or Maine—cats can hunt to their hearts' content with no commentary from humans. But in the world that most of us live in, even small deaths do not go unnoted; and in my little corner of Pennsylvania, the neighbors were starting to talk.

Isabelle next door fretted about the fate of the birds that flock to her multiple feeders. My friend Doris urged me to spare the chipmunks by getting Sasha a bell. Cory up the road weighed in with some circumstantial evidence—the remains of a gray squirrel, its bushy tail still more or less intact—lying suggestively on the path between his house and mine like a smoking gun. And I had qualms of my own.

Was it natural, I wondered, for a cat to bag critter after critter, day after day, and to do it with such ease and aplomb? Moreover, did he have to look so unabashedly triumphant about it? I'm reminded of the day I was roused by the piercing caw of bluejays right outside the living-room window. I went to the door to find Sasha hunkered down on the path in front of the house with a still-living jay in his jaws, looking for all the world like a silent-movie villain—all cheerful malice—as he ties the heroine to the railroad tracks.

Five or six birds, a Greek chorus with feathers, were shrieking their outrage in the trees on either side of him, and Sasha was lucky they didn't launch a dive-bombing counteroffensive. The spring after Tigger joined the household, a group of these big tough birds took to hounding the young cat's footsteps whenever he dared to show his face outdoors. If I wanted to know where Tigger was, I had only to listen for the jays. What had he done to provoke such wrath? And who says prey animals are defenseless?

I actually got concerned enough about Sasha's incessant hunting to ask Dr. Dubensky about it.

"He kills an awful lot of critters," I said hesitantly, as if my cat's being a serial killer were a reflection on the way I had raised him. Too much violent TV, too many Twinkies, so to speak.

"Good!" said the vet matter-of-factly as he reached down to stroke Sasha with, it seemed to me, new respect. "That's what cats are supposed to do."

I felt reassured enough by this exchange to veto Doris's suggestion that I rob Sasha of his potency, as Delilah did Samson, by belling him. Although I had doubts of my own about Sasha's hunting exploits (inconveniently mixed with proprietary pride), I couldn't bear to keep him in a state of perpetual frustration with a bell. In the lethal contest of which Sasha was a part, it didn't make sense to side with anonymous critters over a member of my own household. When you live with a hunting cat you get a front-row seat on the Darwinian struggle for survival, and sometimes you can't help but root for the fittest.

*       *       *

I first began to suspect that I needed to reexamine my thinking on the subject of predation the day Doris and I rescued a bunny, which happened to be firmly clamped in Sasha's jaws at the time. There's nothing cuter than a baby rabbit (perhaps nothing tastier from a feline point of view?). This one was soft and brown and trembling, and about the size of the palm of my hand—so adorable that Doris and I chased Sasha around the yard until we forced him to accede to the iron rule of the jungle and relinquish his prey to two predators larger than himself. Sasha opened his mouth and out the rabbit came, like Jonah released from the whale. And as glad as I was to have saved the little guy, the incident touched off an inner debate.

Would Doris and I have interfered, I wondered, if Sasha had come home carrying a mouse or a rat or a vole? If not, why not? Are those animals more expendable than a baby bunny because they're not as cute? Must a creature look like a Beatrix Potter painting to gain our sympathy? Or do we think less of them because they're "pests"? Well, bunnies are pests, too. They're rodents. They grow up to be rabbits. And rabbits, as anyone who lives in the country can tell you, can demolish a garden, fast.

Perhaps we devalue them because we see them as less intelligent, farther from us in consciousness? If that's the measure, then Sasha should rank higher than any of these others. He outsmarts them by a long shot—perhaps by the very fact of having been born, like us, one of nature's nobility: a predator, member in good standing of the top-of-the-food-chain elite. A cat is born to kill, and even a pampered house pet feels the primal pull. He doesn't stop to consider that there's no reason to nail this jay or that baby rabbit because a nice bowl of Meow Mix awaits him at home.

It's that very juncture, of course—the intersection of the cat's domestic virtues and his killer instincts—that is so hard to parse for us humans. The urge to, say, shoot a coyote who's attacking livestock is comprehensible from the viewpoint of a rancher's self-interest. In Darwinian terms, he's a competitor. The impulse is to protect what's ours, to defend the tenuous boundary between the wild life and the civilized in the same way that a farmer hacks away at the forest that keeps threatening to engulf his fields, or my neighbor Cory erects a chickenwire fence around his vegetable garden, an effective if unaesthetic barrier against rabbits and woodchucks and deer. The minute we humans turn our backs, it seems, Nature comes at us wearing her darkest, most chaotic face.

But what are we to think when the dark side is embodied in the trusted, purring friend who curls up contentedly at the foot of our bed every night? Something seems out of kilter here, the dividing line between nature and culture subtly but profoundly askew. Complicating our thinking, perhaps, is a touch of unconscious envy at the cat's swift and guileless use of force, a tactic that's denied to those of us with aspirations to polite society, but which thrills us nonetheless.

        &#10022;    &#10022;    &#10022;

Home exerts a gravitational pull on a cat, for he is as much a citizen of this cozy world as of the harsher one outside its four walls. And so they come home with their kills. Home is the "den," the center of the territory, and a safe place to make a kill—a place where a cat is unlikely to be molested by other predators who would like nothing better than to take away what he's got. The big cats sometimes drag carrion back to home base for this reason, and many a leopard stashing prey in a favorite tree has been grateful he's a more accomplished high-wire artist than the bigger lions are. Observers in Africa often see lions looking up longingly at the high branches of a tree one of the spotted cats is using as a larder.

But in the domestic landscape, the lure of home is coupled with another phenomenon: the fact that cats seem to want human validation for their hunting accomplishments. They like to show us what they've caught, and they always seem eager for a response. (How disappointed they must be, and how dim they must think us, whenever the response is "Ugh!") The conventional wisdom I've heard since I was a little girl is that cats are bringing you a gift and expect to be praised in return. But the animal behaviorist Desmond Morris, in his book *Catwatching*, offers an alternative theory. Morris believes that just as a mother cat brings home live (or half-dead) prey for her kittens to practice on, so domestic cats are hoping to tutor their humans in the sport they find so engaging.

If this is so, then Sasha, for one, is a most ungenerous teacher. He once slipped inside with a live chipmunk in his mouth and growled threateningly when a friend—having armed himself with the heavy suede work gloves I use at the fireplace—tried to take the animal away. The message was utterly clear: "This is *my* chipmunk, don't you dare touch it. If you want one of your own, you'd best go out and catch it."

My own theory is that cats bring home their catches in an effort at communication—as a primitive form of language, if you will. "Why, when something important happens to you, do you feel compelled to tell someone else about it?" asks Roger Schank in *Tell Me a Story*, his book on language. "Even people who are reticent to talk about themselves can't help telling others about events significant to them. It's as if nothing has happened until an event is made explicit in language." For cats, we humans are very significant others; perhaps they share the important news that they have had a successful hunt simply so that we may bear witness.

In the early days of our life in the country, when he was still fine-tuning his predatory skills, Sasha brought even the smallest, most inconsequential critters back to our door to show me—mice the size of hickory nuts and tiny, sightless voles with pointed snouts. Nowadays, though, he usually doesn't bother, although I know he still hunts the prosaic variety of prey, for I see him in the yard pouncing on these animals or carrying them about. And sometimes, as with the bird skull, I find the remains in my garden, where the cats like to toss, and occasionally half-bury, their booty.

But these critters are old news. Nowadays, like a numismatist chasing the rarest collectibles—a steel penny, a three-legged-buffalo nickel—Sasha brings home only the exotic and unusual specimens he finds. A tree frog, a neon-pink salamander, the baby rabbit that Doris and I took pity on and traitorously released, to my cat's chagrin.

One time I met Sasha out on the path with a green and yellow garter snake suspended horizontally from his mouth like a living handlebar mustache. Sasha had picked the snake up precisely at midpoint, and its equilateral front and rear sections were curling backward and forward, Medusa-like, around his head. Its little forked tongue flicked impatiently in and out.

The cat loped toward me with a particularly avid look on his face—I'm tempted to say he was smiling, so great was his enjoyment of this interesting new experience. He tossed the trophy down at my feet, then threw himself down beside it, the better to bat at the thing as it wriggled about like the pieces of ribbon I would dangle for him to play with when he was a kitten.

The snake endured being tossed in the air and pounced on for a while, and then wisely chose to play dead. Getting no further reaction from his victim, Sasha soon grew bored and stalked off to look for new adventures—whereupon the snake slithered away, apparently none the worse for wear. In drawing me into this and other episodes of his predatory education, Sasha is sharing his world with me, offering a privileged peek at what it means to be a hunting cat.

*     *     *

One day, at just around sunset, I was taking a walk with Sasha when I saw up ahead of us, marching toward Cory's lush vegetable garden, a large brown rabbit too strong and mature looking—too wild—to have stepped from the pages of Beatrix Potter. Perhaps, I fantasized, it was the same rabbit, now grown, that Doris and I had pried from Sasha's jaws just a couple of months before—a vegetarian predator come back to vex my neighbor and terrorize his plants.

Wondering how my cat would react to a prey animal that probably weighed more than he did, I pointed the rabbit out to Sasha, who was a few paces behind me sniffing at a seemingly innocuous patch of weeds that for some reason (territorial markings by another cat?) he found deeply compelling.

As soon as Sasha spotted the rabbit, he dropped into his elongated, aerodynamic hunting crouch, forming a sleek, taut, tensely vibrating line from outstretched head to tip of outstretched tail. Then he paused and looked up at me, as if unsure whether to proceed. It may be my imagination, but it seemed as if only upon seeing that I had an interest in the chase did the cat spring into action.

The rabbit, of course, was far too fast for him. Sasha loped after it for about ten yards, but didn't seem serious about the pursuit. He watched it vanish into the woods near the Kroen-

ers' house, where Buddy lives, then turned around and sauntered back to me with tail upraised as if to say, "Now can we
continue our walk?"

The world is divided into two camps, predator and prey,
but that's not the same as saying that one side is invincible
while the other side rolls over and plays dead. Nature has given
to each in equal measure. Sasha has claws and fangs, the rabbit
size and speed, and the match between the two is not at all un-
equal.

One of the services that scientists studying animals in the
wild perform is to demystify these creatures for us, unraveling
the myths and metaphors human beings may have concocted
through painstaking observations and analysis. In reading
Cynthia Moss's account of various studies of the big cats of
Africa in *Portraits in the Wild,* for example, I was struck by how
much hard work it takes to be a successful predator, and how
much frustration must be endured.

Lions would seem to have an enviable life, sleeping and laz-
ing around for a good part of the day and knocking off an antelope or two when it's time for dinner. Actually, though, hunting takes immense amounts of energy, effort, and guile, and the
cats must make repeated attempts at it in the course of a day's
work before they finally catch something substantial enough to
feed a group of three-hundred-pound carnivores.

Even the most vulnerable-looking antelope has developed
extremely effective anti-predator devices. Tiny ones like the
dik-dik are blessed with lightning speed. Big ones like the
eland find safety in numbers. The midsize impala bursts ten
feet into the air on sighting a predator, and a herd of these animals popping off in all directions, like corks from a case of ex-
ploding champagne bottles, so confuses a lion that she may not
be able to single out one individual for a hit.

The balance, says Moss, "is often in favor of the prey"; a

lone lioness succeeds "in only 17 percent of her hunting attempts." The hit ratio rises when the lions hunt in groups, but it's still no walk in the park.

*      *      *

The fact that my cats, too, are far from invincible hunters was brought home to me—literally—not long ago, when Charcoal darted past me on a beautiful summer day and tore into the house with a live chipmunk in his mouth. He dropped it on the living-room rug and looked up at me with a self-satisfied smile—"Aren't I clever?" he seemed to be asking—whereupon the chipmunk took off on a survivalist adventure that was to keep all of us hopping for the next forty-eight hours.

Chipmunks are fast. Real fast. Too fast, as it turned out, for Charcoal. Like a cartoon cat-villian and with about as much success, he chased it around the living room and dining room, thumping heavily against the furniture as he went. No matter. Like a dik-dik outsprinting a lion, the chipmunk repeatedly evaded recapture over the course of that first afternoon in my house, and he managed to find hideouts neither the cats nor I could discover in between his desperate breaks for freedom.

Day passed into evening, and evening into morning, and still the chipmunk survived. I began to wonder if I'd ever get rid of him—can you domesticate a chipmunk?—and wavered between hoping the cats would catch him and get it over with, and wanting to set him free. As for my cats, I'm sorry to report that they failed to empathize in any way with my predicament. Not in the face of feline bread and circuses.

On the second day, Charcoal cornered the chipmunk at one point behind a sturdy, log-based plant stand in the dining room, the chipmunk crying out his distress—or his rage—in a wave of high-pitched squirrelly chirps. I locked the cat in the bathroom to keep him out of the way and found two big baskets, which I set down at either end of the plant stand's base with the openings facing inward. My hope was that the chipmunk would dash into one of them. I would then cover one basket with the other, creating a kind of ad hoc wicker hamper in which to tote him outside.

But the chipmunk refused to budge, even when I prodded him with my glove-tipped finger. Finally he edged into one of the baskets, but panicked when I upended it, escaping once more into the wilderness that was my house.

I didn't see the chipmunk again all day. But that night the ever vigilant Sasha stationed himself by one of the grates that are built into either side of my fireplace and lay staring into its depths as if it were Aladdin's magic cave, pawing between the bars from time to time. From this I deduced that the chipmunk was camping out in there. By now I was feeling sorry for the tenacious little creature, who hadn't had food or water for over a day (unless he managed to sneak some out of the cats' bowls when they weren't looking). Along with compassion, though, was self-interest: the last thing I wanted was for the chipmunk to expire in the unseen interstices of my fireplace.

And so I set up my own version of a Haveaheart trap. I got out a cardboard box, set it on its side, and put a small bowl of water and a scattering of raisin bran inside. (I didn't know if chipmunks liked raisin bran, but it was the only thing I had in the house that seemed remotely appropriate.) I edged this contraption up to the fireplace, angled it to place the opening of the box over the grate, and taped the flaps down securely with shiny silver duct tape. The only place the chipmunk could now move, or so I thought, was between grate and box. My plan was to rip off the tape, upend the box, and close the flaps as soon as I heard claws scrabbling on cardboard. Then I would release the beast outdoors—far, far away from my house.

All that evening there was no sign of life, in the box or behind the grate. Finally I gave up and went to bed, and I awoke early the next morning to the sound of a chase. Looking down from the loft bedroom, I could see that the wily chipmunk had somehow gotten by the trap—only to emerge into the daylight of the living room and find himself face to face with Sasha. All at once the cat caught him by the scruff of his neck and began parading around the living room, head raised high and chest puffed out, like a general showing off his medals in a victory parade. To my dismay, he then trotted smartly up the stairs to the bedroom and dropped his trophy at my feet.

The chipmunk tore off once more, tumbling down the stairs with two cats now in antic pursuit. He wheeled across the living room, as fast and erratic as my nephew's remote-control racecar, then crossed the hall and dashed into the bathroom. I moved in one step ahead of the cats and shut the bathroom door in their faces. Then I put both cats outside and called the helpful folks at the local office of the National Park Service to find out what to do.

Just open the window, they said, the chipmunk will find his way out. I was dubious that a chipmunk could scale sheer walls to reach the window, which is about four feet off the floor. But when I went into the bathroom a moment later to dutifully re-move the screens, the little fellow sat perched in my sink, clearly in search of an exit. He looked as chipper as could be— the very definition of bright-eyed and bushy-tailed—despite the travails of the previous two days. Never underestimate the power of a chipmunk.

I cranked open both sides of the casement window as wide as they would go, lifted out the screens, and closed the door behind me. The next time I checked, an hour or so later, the doughty chipmunk had departed, just as the Park Rangers promised he would. It's amazing that Charcoal managed to nab this *Uber* chipmunk in the first place, and instructive to note that once he did, neither he nor Sasha was able to kill it. The animals they do kill, I assume, are either less resourceful or more vulnerable than this one.

*     *     *

I've never tracked Sasha throughout the day as a scientist would to record how many kills he makes versus how many attempts. One estimate I've read is that cats miss two times out of three. As our resident chipmunk proved, Chip and Dale—and bird and mouse and rabbit—are as well equipped with anti-predator defenses as any eland or impala.

Still, my cats do make kills—daily, in the warm months— and thus they have an impact on the local ecosystem, the neighborhood cycle of life and death. Just what that impact might be, however, sinister or otherwise, is open to discussion.

A couple of British biologists who conducted a systematic study of feline predation in a small Bedfordshire village a few years ago concluded that house cats are the most successful predators around, beating owls and foxes handily in number of kills. The 78 village cats they studied nailed 1,100 critters—64 percent of them rodents—in a year, with a few inept cats contributing little or nothing to the total and a few supercats downing 100 animals apiece. (Those totals represent just the prey the cats dragged home to their owners, who obligingly stashed the remains in little plastic freezer bags until the scientists fetched them; undoubtedly more than a few catches were consumed on the spot or got left behind in the woods.)

Extrapolating their findings to the estimated total domestic cat population of the United Kingdom, the researchers figure that house cats account for "about seventy million deaths" a year in Britain. That is, indeed, a body count to reckon with. But what does it really mean? The scientists offer up their computations but leave ethical evaluation to the reader.

While statistics are not my strong suit, I decided to try some number crunching based on their results.

Dividing 1,100 corpses by 78 cats reveals that the average kill ratio of the cats in the study is a mere 14 animals per year apiece, 9 of which would be rodents based on the two-thirds ratio the scientists cited. Let's assume for argument's sake that all three of my cats—Sasha, Charcoal, and Tigger, who has proven to be a formidable hunter in his own right—make that average. That's forty-two small deaths in our little neighborhood per year, twenty-seven of them mice, voles, chipmunks, or other rodents, the rest birds and "other," like Sasha's snake and salamander.

Sorry, but I've seen the evidence and that just doesn't sound like enough.

So let's up the ante and assume that two of my three cats fall into the scientists' supercat category (I doubt, in terms of odds, that all three would, especially given that Charcoal stays indoors so much). If so, they might jointly bag 200 prey animals a year—say 214, if two cats are aces and the third plugs along at the average pace. Based on the English model, 137 of these kills would be rodents, 77 birds and miscellaneous.

Crunching the numbers yet again to get a daily rate, my three cats combined might be responsible for anywhere from .12 (the U.K. average) to .59 (Terminator II) deaths a day. A worst-case scenario, in other words, of less than one.

I don't mean to make light of the problem that exists in areas where rare or endangered songbirds are falling prey to cats. But all things being equal, is my neighborhood any poorer in diversity of life on account of losing somewhere in the vicinity of one mouse or chipmunk or bird every other day to my cats? Did I unalterably degrade the environment when I introduced cats here?

Or could my cats somehow compensate, in the grand

scheme of things, for the decline in wild predators—the owls and foxes the English researchers compare them with—that inevitably accompanies human habitation? It's interesting to note the biologists found that cats at the wooded edges of town had significantly higher kill ratios than those living in the village center. From this I conclude that factors like human and cat population density—or simple lack of opportunity—might serve as natural checks and balances.

Perhaps the rodent population here would undergo an alarming, Malthusian growth spurt were it not for my cats, just as our white-tailed deer have soared to numbers that would stun the original inhabitants of these parts, now that none but human predators (and their cars) remain.

Perhaps my cats enhance the populations they hunt by ferreting out the weaklings, leaving only the most robust individuals, like the indomitable chipmunk in the bathroom sink, to pass on their genetic material.

Perhaps my cats are just being cats, acting out parts in a tale that predates the human drama.

And perhaps my own consternation at the sometimes grisly spectacles intrinsic to life with a predator springs not from an affinity for nature's littlest creatures, but from bewilderment in the face of these constant reminders that "nature" is not synonymous with benign beauty, the way I might like it to be. My cats keep informing me that it's also a metaphysical drama of life and death in their rawest, least civilized forms.

❖    ❖    ❖

By now my cats have trained me, largely through repetition, to appreciate their hunting, in the way that one appreciates mastery wherever it is found; to be tolerant, if not exactly enthusiastic. Sometimes I'm actually grateful to them. I need never set a mousetrap, as my neighbors do—no mouse would be foolish enough to set up housekeeping at my place. The destructive red squirrels pick other people's attics to invade; the voles burrow in other people's gardens, and the birds leave my strawberries alone. One time a bat got into the house. Sasha caught it and held it immobile long enough for a man friend to scoop it up in an empty coffee can and release it outside.

In deference to this lesson, I kept the melancholy little bird skull that I dug up out of the garden. It sits on the mantel in a pottery bowl of robin's egg blue that's filled with curiosities of nature: seashells, a fossil or two, the skeleton of a seahorse. In the midst of life, death.

My cats may not appreciate the gesture, but I do.

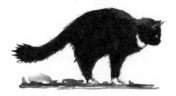

# 12  Decoding the Litter Box

I doubt if Al Gore had Kitty Litter in mind when he began promoting the information superhighway, but that was the topic being discussed not long ago on one of CompuServe's electronic bulletin boards. GO PETS is what you type to get into the network's Animal Forum, whereupon a menu comes up on your computer screen offering sixteen special-interest choices, such as Tooth 'n' Claw, The Fire Hydrant, Reptiles/Exotic, and Ask-A-Vet. I always pick Number 4, Cat's Meow, and I dropped in one day to find myself privy to a discussion of scoopable litter.

.  This technological breakthrough in feline hygiene burst upon the cat scene a few years back. I well remember its advent, because a woman I worked with at the time was selling this miracle substance on the side, the way other people sell Amway or Avon, and she came around the office proselytizing. It sounded pretty intriguing, so I bought some. It came not in bags, like regular litter, but in gallon jugs, like bleach. It was different, too, in texture. An extremely fine-grained, almost silky, sand, this stuff was yin to clay-based litter's yang.

Now widely sold under a dizzying variety of brand names, scoopable litter works by "trapping" liquids upon contact, so instead of diffusing through the box and making the whole thing reek of ammonia, cat puddles stay put. They combine with the siltlike substance to form discrete little balls, or chunks, that can be lifted out and discarded the same way you clean out (pardon the expression) solid wastes. The rest of the litter remains unsullied and therefore lasts for quite a while—a couple of weeks or even longer, if only one cat is using the box—without needing to be changed.

This trail-blazing litter held all the glittering promise of any other revolutionary new product, penicillin, say, or Velcro. It represented a quantum leap forward for the cat litter industry, and for the legions of those who have cats. Scoopable litter would lighten our burdens, eliminate muss and fuss, save time, change our lives. It wasn't a cure for the common cold, but for cat owners it was the next best thing. Ask anyone who cleans out a litter box once a week.

But as the old saying goes, every stick has two ends, and scoopable litter is no exception.

"I see you use the scoopable litter," wrote Davie, as he joined the electronic discussion. "I take it this is the kind that clumps into little balls. I tried it once or twice, but the sandlike substance it's made from would stick to the bottoms of all the little fuzzy paws in the house and get tracked all over the house." Davie suggested an alternative, a product called Good

Mews that "seems to be made from rolled paper. It looks just like rabbit pellets. It controls the odor really well, stays in the box, is inexpensive, and the cats seem to like it."

Davie was not alone with the tracking problem. "I also got the entire Sahara in silicon grit all over the rug," Helen empathized. "The kittens were extremely distressed about having the litter stick to their paws. You should have seen their widdie faces!" One participant puts sisal mats around the litter box so her cat can wipe its feet.

Aside from tracking, another difficulty posed by scoopable litter is hardware-related: what kind of scoop to scoop with. "I know of one couple who had a running feud about which was better for scooping clumpable litter, the metal scoops or the plastic ones," wrote Gayle. "I have had clumps break with both kinds, but I've also broken the plastic ones several times trying to remove particularly large clumps. We have a metal one now that can handle the HD [heavy-duty formula]."

Of preeminent concern is getting cats, conservatives that they are, to accept a new kind of litter. "Our cats viewed the scoopable stuff with great suspicion," wrote Janet, "and did a lot of scooping themselves—right out onto the floor."

Ah yes, the "dig-to-China school of litter maintenance," replied Martha, who copes with this habit by using steep-sided boxes, such as dishpans. Another correspondent suggested covered litter boxes—the kind that look like cat-size Conestoga wagons—as a solution for steamshovel cats. But cats don't always like them. "Our cats use the snap-on lids as a place on which to deposit their, ah, creations," said Janet, with a delicacy worthy of Henry James.

My own experience with the scoopable litter was inconclusive. It seemed like a good product and I've bought more of it since. I also buy the clay litter. It's just not an urgent issue any more, because now that I live in the country, my cats disdain their boxes except in the case of dire need (e.g., when I go away and they're stuck inside) or atrocious weather (Siberian cold snaps, monsoons). They much prefer going outdoors, the way God intended, and only rarely do I ever have to deal with their, ah, creations.

Not only that, but among its many charms my house boasts a half-bath downstairs, off my workroom, and this is where the cat boxes are kept. The line is drawn: I have my bathroom and you cats have yours. Hallelujah! No more litter on the bathmat in the mornings! Moving to Pennsylvania has thus enhanced my quality of life in more ways than I ever imagined possible when I bought my house.

*     *     *

I do keep the litter boxes clean and change them as needed, however. And in doing so I've noticed an interesting piece of behavior on Sasha's part that makes me think there's more to the cat litter question than meets the eye.

An intensely curious cat who takes an active role in the running of the household, Sasha finds it a deeply meaningful event whenever I perform the litter rites: dumping the contents of the three low-sided plastic pans, one beige, one turquoise, and the other one lime green, into a big trash bag, rinsing them out, and then refilling them—an avalanche of nice clean litter whooshing resoundingly from the bag or jug of whatever brand I hauled home from the supermarket that week.

The instant that Box Number 1 has been filled, Sasha climbs into it. He turns to face me, his back legs splayed against the sides of the box and an earnest look on his face. Then he pees. Upon completion, he turns and sniffs at what he's done as if to see that it's satisfactory. Apparently it is, and so he briskly scratches at the litter beside it until the puddle is nicely covered. He then climbs into each of the other boxes in turn, but by now he has nothing left with which to christen them and must satisfy himself with pawing.

Now, Sasha can relieve himself pretty much any time he wants to simply by going outdoors, so I know he hasn't been waiting uncomfortably for opportunity to present itself in the form of a clean litter box. (Indoor cats sometimes will, so scrupulous are cats about the state of the latrine; I know the feeling every time I go into a gas station rest room.) Instead, it appears that Sasha is translating the same territorial marking behavior he practices outdoors, or a version thereof, to the litter box inside. Like Kilroy, he finds it necessary to leave behind a message testifying that "I was here."

◆   ◆   ◆

Comparatively speaking, the question of bathroom habits is simple for a cat. You buy him a box, you fill it with litter, he uses it. Even the littlest kitten knows how, and there's no need for the kind of extended training that puppies (or babies) require. Yet whenever you "civilize" a biological function, especially one so central as elimination, you've set the stage for drama. The box is a sanctum sanctorum where a cat may attend to his organic needs, and many cats are very fussy indeed about its care and maintenance.

I have three litter boxes, one per cat, but as best as I can tell my cats aren't proprietary and will indiscriminately use any of them when the need arises. However, some cats—Mimsy and Jean Arthur were among them—insist on a box of one's own. One participant in the CompuServe colloquy said he had six boxes for nine cats, but he didn't detail how the cats apportion them among themselves.

While Sasha will share a litter box with his two housemates, he won't share with just anyone. During the short spell a few years ago that he spent as an "only" cat—after Mimsy and Jean Arthur had died, but before Charcoal moved in full time—Sasha stayed at my friend Linda's for a week when I went away on vacation. Linda had a litter box from her cat, Max, who had died a while before, so I didn't bother bringing Sasha's pan from home; just a bag of fresh litter. But I found out upon my return that my normally well-behaved cat had refused to use the box, opting instead for the bathtub in the laundry room.

Did Sasha sniff on the box the ghostly vestiges of Max? Did he fear the rightful owner would show up to complain? Or was Sasha gripped with anxiety to find himself plunked down amid strangers in a place where nothing—not even the litter box—bore his own familiar scent? Whatever the answer, it suggests that a breach of litter box taboos must be a grave affront indeed among cats.

Happily, Linda quickly realized what the problem was and cut down a territorially neutral cardboard box from the supermarket, which she then filled with litter. Sasha gratefully accepted the compromise, and Linda has never held his litter box lapse against him.

All too often, however, solutions are not this easy to find, and the litter box becomes a site fraught with tribulation for both owner and cat. A cat for whom, heretofore, cleanliness has been next to godliness will suddenly start to have "accidents," which we humans must try to decode. Physical ailment? Emotional upset? Simple dislike of a new kind of litter?

Such questions involved me for all of the fifteen years I lived with Jean Arthur, who for reasons I never fully understood found the litter box to be a place of hazard and dread. As a kitten, she would sometimes use the box and sometimes back into a corner to pee, a terrorized look on her face. What was so scary? I never knew. Box use and non-use didn't seem to correlate to anything going on in her environment at the moment; the demons arose from within.

She got better as she got older, but throughout her lifetime this sensitive little cat would promptly forget how to use the box whenever she went through an upsetting experience—anything from a major life change, like moving, to, who knows, the sudden appearance of a dust mote or the convergence of Mercury and Venus. She was also prone to urinary-tract infections, which could have been either chicken or egg in terms of her litter box aversion. Either way, they didn't help.

At one point, in one apartment, she was using the bathtub as a litter box the same way Sasha did at Linda's. I've since been informed that tub use sometimes signals the onset of an infection. At the time, though, I had just been told that scattering fresh onion slices wherever the cat has taken to peeing is a good deterrent, since cats don't like strong odors, and so I cut up onions by the bushelful. They were no match for Jean Arthur. She continued to do her business in the tub, right on top of the onions, and I quickly gave up on this tactic.

◇   ◆   ◆

As easily as most cats take to using a box, its presence in the house is perhaps a tad confusing for them. Cats don't respect the distinction between outdoors and in under the best of circumstances; it's all just habitat to them. When Sasha perches atop one of the tall bookcases that line one wall of my workroom, he might just as well be surveying the countryside from some rocky crag. When he chases one of the other cats off the bed or the couch, he's defending territory in much the same way that he does outdoors. When he comes to the door with a creature in his teeth, he'd like nothing better than to get my okay to tear it apart in the house. (This is especially true if it's raining, when the shelter of the living room is obviously preferable to the dank, dripping yard.) How much more ambiguous it all becomes when we bring the outdoors in in the form of dirt, which is all litter is, no matter how fetchingly packaged.

Plants are another item with dual citizenship, so I guess I shouldn't have been as astounded as I was last December when Sasha backed into his "marking" posture in front of the Christmas tree, raised his tail, and gave it a little spritz. He's never done anything of the kind in the house before. But then, it was I who set the stage for confusion by bringing in a live blue spruce in a pot instead of the standard cut tree in a tippy metal holder. I won't think twice if Sasha marks this tree now that I've planted it outdoors. But at the time I didn't appreciate his failure to grasp its symbolic function.

It's very much the same with a garden. To us humans a garden represents an extension of the domestic interior transplanted out of doors, our personal experiment (successful or otherwise) in taming nature and shaping it to our will. But what seems to us a civilized, or semi-civilized, space is, to to my cats, nothing more than dirt, plants, and shrubs, indistinguishable from the scrub along the hillside or the ragged woods in the vacant lot across from Doris's house.

Basically my cats are right. A garden isn't anything more than dirt, plants, and shrubs, except that it's dirt, plants, and shrubs selected, tended—and thus given meaning—by us. So last summer it was no time for rejoicing when one or more of my cats (I was never sure who the culprit was) decided that a particular patch of dirt—otherwise known as Isabelle's garden—would make a great latrine. The nice soft soil, so lovingly worked by this eightysomething woman, must have felt soothing on the paws. Repellent spray and odiferous pellets purchased at the hardware store dissuaded them of this idea, and they eventually moved on to a less obtrusive spot.

Sometimes it's not our cats who blur the boundaries and mix the metaphors, but us. Since nothing is more biodegradable than dirt, an environmentally conscious friend of mine has taken to disposing of used cat litter outside rather than dumping it in the trash. Once a week she scatters the contents of her cat's box here and there in little piles toward the rear of her large lot, or mounds it fetishistically around tree trunks. Her cat, a smoky gray female named Sweetpea, mainly stays indoors. But thanks to her owner's efforts, her territory is marked as efficiently as if she were to go outside and do it herself.

Simply by dint of being animals, cats are close to their own organic nature in a way that we humans are not. It's no wonder, then, that they're not at all reluctant to admit to an abiding interest in both their litter boxes and the deposits they leave behind there. It's also unsurprising that they may use the box—or fail to—as a soapbox, conveying stress, anger, or other messages by process of elimination, as it were. Sometimes these communiques seem intentional, their symbolism consciously chosen. Consider the examples of Venus and Jupiter (who are unrelated, although their names make it sound like they should be).

Venus was an abused stray rescued by a woman who already had two cats, one of whom nervily availed himself of the litter box that had been set up specifically for Venus. But this little black and white cat retaliated in kind. In an inspired move, she walked over to the resident cat's water bowl and peed in it— poetic justice, to be sure.

As for Jupiter, this gray and white cat found himself getting locked up daily in an oversize wire cage one Christmas season, his owners' way of keeping him from demolishing the decorations. Besides the tree, always an irresistible target for a young cat, these included an elaborate model racecar exhibit, complete with a network of interconnecting tracks and assorted small buildings and scenery. The previous Christmas, Jupiter's owners had come home from work each day to find the diorama dismantled, cars and tracks and tiny bits of city scattered all over the apartment as if King Kong had passed through while they were out.

They tried locking the cat in the bathroom—the only room with a door in their open-plan apartment—during the hours they were not at home, but he was unhappy there. And so they acquired the cage, which they outfitted with food and water dishes, a big plush cushion for the cat to nap on, and, for obvious reasons, a litter pan.

But Jupiter didn't like the cage. And he let his jailers know it by dumping a great big pile of turds not in his litter box, which he had never failed to use before, but right on top of the pillow on which he was supposed to sleep—a succinct, even eloquent, statement, given the limited range of expression available to him under the circumstances. We humans do the same thing, albeit symbolically, when we advertise our anger with a loud exclamation of *"Merde!"* or "I'm pissed!"

For what it's worth, the couple ultimately devised a creative solution to their problem. They bought a thick, bright red cat sweater that was just a wee bit too snug for Jupiter and dressed him up in it every morning. It left him ambulatory—but without enough freedom of movement to make flying leaps onto the racecar display or the tree. Despite an unfortunate subtext of feline straitjacket, the sweater made Jupiter a lot happier than the despised and defiled cage.

I thought of Venus and Jupiter recently when my neighbor across the way—a very old, very unpleasant woman who is deservedly friendless in the neighborhood—took to throwing her cocker spaniel's droppings out onto the well-traveled foot path in front of her house. Requests to cease didn't help, nor did one neighbor's eye-for-an-eye approach (he scooped the doggie do off the path and threw it back into the old woman's yard).

Finally I went over to her with a small plastic garbage can and an offer to empty it weekly, on garbage day, if only she would use it. Much to my surprise, she agreed. In fact, not only was she not insulted by my intrusion, she actually seemed delighted with the attention. And like a canny congressman cutting a deal, she used the implied threat of noncompliance to get me to agree to pick up her mail every day, too, from the mailboxes out on the road.

It dawned on me then that her antisocial gesture was not a simple lack of consideration, but a statement of some sort, no less emphatic than Jupiter's—an "Up yours!", perhaps, to all of us who so thoroughly ignored her. Turning the path into a minefield of dog droppings made it impossible to ignore her. Curse her we might as we picked our way down the road or scraped off our shoes afterward. But perhaps it is better to be cursed than forgotten.

❖   ❖   ❖

You'd be surprised at the number of people who told me, when I mentioned I was working on this chapter, that cats can be trained to use the toilet. None of my informants actually knew of any who had been, or of any cat owners who had tried. Still, they insisted, the potty is the next frontier. Imagine! No more boxes to clean and change. No more litter, scoopable or otherwise, to buy.

I had my doubts. If cats are suspicious of a new kind of litter, as the CompuServe discussion suggested, would they take at all kindly to no litter at all? How would they satisfy the innate urge to scratch and cover, given that porcelain doesn't offer the same tactile rewards as dirt? Moreover, what about logistics? How would you negotiate the positioning of the toilet seat (He says up, She says down) if Fluffy were to join Mom and Dad in the bathroom?

Upon further questioning, it seemed that everyone's knowledge of feline toilet training began and ended with an episode of *Designing Women* on TV, in which Jan Hooks kept everyone else in the cast from entering the office rest room because she was training her cat. The regimen apparently involves first resting the litter box, which at this point is filled in the traditional way, on top of the toilet seat to get the cat accustomed to going about her business up there. Eventually you remove the box, and Fluff—now conditioned to associate toilet seat with elimination—takes that next radical step. All the cat owner need do is flush.

Uh huh.

Still, it might not be as unnatural as it would seem at first blush for a cat to prefer water to earth for her most elemental of needs. Not if you consider the jaguarundi, a slim, grayish, long-tailed native of Central and South America. That this cat demands a watery latrine is one of the esoteric facts I picked up from a collection of essays called *Man and Beast: Revisited,* based on a conference some years back at the Smithsonian Institution. Among the more intriguing articles was a memoir by Michael H. Robinson, the director of the National Zoo in Washington, D.C., of his fieldwork in Panama, where he and his wife kept a jaguarundi. Her name was Jackie, and she had no interest in traditional litter.

"By day, [she] simply urinated on the tiled house floor," Robinson writes. "This was perfectly acceptable, since it could be easily mopped up and left no permanent effect." Nighttime was tougher, because Jackie "slept in a warm hollow at the small of my back and . . . I woke frequently to a warm glow," as Robinson delicately puts it.

This tolerant scientist found the key to the problem by accident. "One day," he says, "[Jackie] stood in the raccoon's water manipulation tray and used that; afterward we provided a water-filled cat box."

I hate to think how the raccoon must have felt; perhaps as

outdone as the cat whose water dish Venus once despoiled. But it's gratifying to hear that this wild, or semi-wild, feline found a way to communicate to her human housemates the precise nature of her needs. Perhaps she's a candidate for training on the loo. Maybe she could even learn to flush.

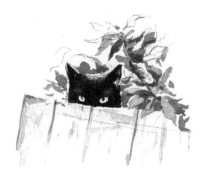

# 13  The Red-Headed League

There's something about autumn and cats. Sasha entered my life in the month of October and Charcoal showed up on a fall day two years later, so it seemed only natural that the third member of the household should arrive in autumn, too. Especially since his coloring matched the season.

He was a small orange kitten—about four months old, the vet guessed—with fur complexly patterned in rich, dense, tone-on-tone stripes and swirls that made his coat look like watered silk. I say orange for convenience sake, but it was actually a subtler mix: peach and gold and amber, overlaid with a spicy ginger that in some lights seemed russet or cinnamon—the colors of Florentine rooftops, or October in Vermont. The only deviation from this burnished palette was a white chin and whiskers. His eyes were copper, the same as his fur, and his nose and paw pads were salmon pink, like a newly unwrapped piece of bubble gum.

Some cats get adopted because of their spunk. They grab your attention and charm you into taking them home. Sasha was this kind of cat. Others move in like squatters and never leave—witness Charcoal. A third variety have a hard-luck story to tell. They're cats who need to be rescued, and this was the case with Tigger.

It was a late September weekend a year and a half ago, and my mother and my cousin Karen were visiting from New England. The three of us were browsing that warm Sunday afternoon at the local flea market—all too apt, as it turned out, given that the kitten we were about to find there was loaded with real fleas—when I left them momentarily to get something out of the car. That's when I spotted him.

He was sitting by himself in the backseat of a beat-up Chevy. He looked pathetic and unwell, and was mewing quietly to himself as if too weak to stage a bigger ruckus—the picture of despondency. I stopped to look, and was wiggling a finger through the partially open car window in an attempt to get the kitten's attention when I was startled by the sudden appearance of a dark-haired boy of eleven or twelve.

"Do you want him?" the boy asked, and in one motion he opened the car door, scooped up the kitten, and handed him over to me, like a salesman fetching an item from a display case.

The boy and his parents and brother had rescued the cat, he explained, from a group of little boys in their neighborhood who were mistreating him. The boy was certain the kitten was a stray; he had seen him before, knocking around people's backyards. He thought that if he kept the cat he might name him Butterscotch, which seemed wholly inappropriate to me, for it suggested frivolity and sugary-good times whereas the kitten himself did not. But it would be best, the boy continued, if he could find the cat a home, for his family already had five cats, a number of kittens, and a couple of dogs, too.

The boy's parents had by now shown up to verify his story—and so had my mother and cousin, who were cooing over the little redhead nestled wearily in my arms. Every once in a while he leaned back to look pleadingly into my eyes, and he opened his mouth in a silent meow.

I wasn't in the market for another cat, hadn't gone out looking for one. And based on the uproar that ensued when I brought Sasha home to live with Mimsy and Jean Arthur so many years before, I was convinced the number three was cursed when it came to feline population count. Adding a small red kitten to the family didn't seem like a very good idea.

"I think I'll call him Tiger," I said.

"Tigger," my cousin amended. And so Tigger he became.

* * *

Everyone has a story about how they met their cat—the fateful serendipity, the harmonic convergence of place and time, that brought cat and human together. "It was a dark and stormy night," or, "In the beginning was the cat," or, "One autumn day at the flea market. . . ."

These stories make compelling narratives, for the tale of how we turned a scared and scrawny creature such as Tigger was into a sleek, well-loved, contented cat reflects back on the teller, a snapshot of our good intentions. There's a pride in it not unlike the pride that a farmer must feel when he looks on a new crop of piglets or witnesses the birth of a colt—a proprietary joy in being the one to provide an environment in which another may prosper.

The responsibility of caring for this Other calls up something in us—altruism, perhaps, or fellow feeling, a wish to do the right thing. And for rescued cats everywhere, the right thing begins with a trip to the vet, which is where Karen, my mother, the kitten, and I proceeded the very next day.

Tigger had spent the previous night in the bigger of my two cat carriers. This sturdy, beige plastic contraption is large enough for two cats to comfortably travel in, so for one small kitten it was the equivalent of a studio apartment in Manhattan. Tigger seemed to feel safe in its cavelike depths, shielded from the outside world in general and from two (possibly hostile) big black cats in particular. Sasha and Charcoal could sniff something fishy in the air, but with Tigger locked away out of sight they couldn't quite put a paw on what it was.

He drank immense amounts of water—clearly, he had become dehydrated over the course of this stressful day—but turned down cat food, dry or canned. All Tigger wanted was to sleep. He plunked himself down on the towel I had placed in the carrier for him and sank gratefully into deep, restorative unconsciousness.

The next morning he looked a little perkier. He mewed to let us know he needed to come out and use the litter box, then ate and drank a bit before getting nudged back into the carrier for the trip to Dr. Dubensky's.

"I don't know, Jackie, he doesn't look good," said the vet, who quickly diagnosed an infestation of fleas, probable anemia (which follows, for fleas can suck a kitten dry), worms, and an upper respiratory infection. He thought it likely there were other problems lurking beneath these.

"I give him a fifty-fifty chance," the vet said soberly, and he sent me home with assorted medication plus firm instructions to keep the kitten in quarantine for the next three weeks lest he pass any diseases on to Sasha and Charcoal.

Distressed as I was about Tigger's iffy prospects, I also felt thoroughly chastened. Whatever had I been thinking in picking up a sickly stray? I had lucked out with Sasha and Charcoal, each of whom joined the household with no ill effects on the other cats who lived with me at the time. But taking in another foundling was like playing Russian roulette. Who knew what he might be carrying? The life of a street cat is nasty, brutish, and short, and I'd never forgive myself if my black cats got sick on account of a red one I barely knew.

It was in a funereal mood that the four of us retraced our route and drove home, where my mother and cousin helped me set Tigger up in the downstairs bathroom—his home for the immediate future. Given the layout of my house, the only other space I could easily close off as a quarantine ward was the loft bedroom and another room leading up to it—the section of house assigned to Mimsy and Jean Arthur during their turf wars with Sasha five or six years earlier. But I had no intention of kicking Sasha and Charcoal out of their usual sleeping spot—my bed—for the sake of one sick kitten, so the downstairs bathroom it was.

Once the big cats' litter boxes were moved out and a new one for Tigger moved in, it turned out to be a pretty good spot, all things considered. It had a window with a windowsill, upon which Tigger would sit and stare contemplatively into the trees. It was large, as bathrooms go, so there was enough room for the kitten to play. And I brought down the cat carrier so he'd have a familiar place to sleep.

My mother and cousin and I de-flead the cat here, washing him in the sink with Shaklee's Basic H cleaning solution (which I prefer to chemical flea shampoos), then combing him with a fine-toothed flea comb to yank out the remaining high-jumpers, which we proceeded remorselessly to drown. Karen, who is a hairdresser by trade, turned the blow-dryer on Tigger as I simultaneously rubbed him down with a towel, and by the time we were finished, the kitten didn't look half bad.

◆      ◆      ◆

Nature must lavish her restorative powers on the young, for it was amazing to see how rapidly Tigger regained his health once he was rid of internal and external parasites and had been treated to a little TLC. So improved was he after a week or so of strict quarantine that the vet judged it safe to let him out of the bathroom whenever the big cats were not at home—which was often, since we were enjoying an exceptionally warm fall that year and the cats spent much of the day outdoors.

I would let them out in the morning, then troop downstairs to feed Tigger and open up the door to his cell. He was well behaved; he didn't charge off for parts unknown, but stayed by my side in the workroom, where he played with the cat toys the big cats had collected over the years, napped, or sat in a window and looked out. I soon came to rely on his company while I worked. He was a nice little fella to have around, albeit more somber than you would expect a small kitten to be.

As soon as Sasha or Charcoal came indoors, back in the bathroom went Tigger (and I washed my hands before I touched them, as Dr. Dubensky had instructed). As soon as they went back outside, I'd again open Tigger's door, and I started to feel like I was living in one of those French farces where lovers are constantly dashing out one door as spouses come in through another.

But as logistically complex as it sounds, the arrangement turned out to be a good way to get the big cats accustomed to a little one, more or less in absentia. Sasha and Charcoal caught glimpses of Tigger through the huge picture window that looks out from the workroom to the deck, which is where they often linger during the day. And they caught his scent when they came inside. Sometimes they would sniff suspiciously or scratch at the locked bathroom door that separated him from them, but they never caught the perpetrator in the act, never encountered him in the flesh. They were like Mr. Jones in the old Bob Dylan song, who knows something is happening but doesn't know what it is.

By the third week, when I began taking Tigger outdoors on the same blue leash that once had so vexed Sasha, they got a good look at him from a distance. So by the time the kitten went back to the vet's for his shots and a feline leukemia test (mercifully, it was negative), he was able to come home with a clean bill of health and plunge into the life of the household without too much further ado. Sasha and Charcoal had gotten used to him by default, and they found nothing very much to object to once he finally materialized in person.

◆　　◆　　◆

It takes a long time to really get to know someone, and Tigger kept reminding me of this fact after taking up residence in my house. With Sasha I had felt an instant affinity, the kind I've experienced on first meeting certain of my friends; he and I were on the same wavelength from day one. As for Charcoal, he was pretty much an open book; he was easy to love, and his character was not hard to fathom. But Tigger was different. I was struck again and again in those early days by how utterly *himself* he was, and how utterly enigmatic. He stared at me solemnly with eyes the color of pennies, and I was never sure what thoughts might lie behind them. It seemed more than passing strange to have opened my door to this alien consciousness and invited it to come on in.

At the same time, it was enchanting having a kitten in the house again—especially one so interesting to look at. There was a universe to discover in Tigger's moiré fur. His markings were pronounced and precise. Neat, tone-on-tone stripes banded his chest and arms, lightning bolts adorned his cheeks, and on his forehead was a stylized "M" like the one that Bean-head had worn. Between his shoulder blades sat a winglike silhouette that the cat books call a butterfly, and viewed from behind, his rump (minus tail) had the markings of an orange watermelon. The points on his muzzle from which the whiskers emerged were darker than the surrounding fur, and looked like freckles. And his color was hard to pin down. Yellow, orange, red—marmalade cat, ginger tom, tiger—Tigger has been called all of these. After living with him for a while I personally settled on plain old "redhead," for as Tigger grew he began to remind me of the young Jimmy Cagney: small, muscled, carrot-topped, and a little too tightly wound.

In the days when Jean Arthur was alive, some friends in Rhode Island happened also to have longhaired gray cats—two of them, Nigel and Willow. Sometimes we compared notes on this feline trio's personality quirks, and although I no longer recall the details of exactly what these consisted of, the similarities were enough for us to invent an imaginary institution called Gray Cat School.

"Willow and Nigel do that too; they must have all learned it at Gray Cat School," my friends would say when I shared some oddity from Jeannie's behavioral repertoire. I never posited a similar "school" for the black cats to which I seem to gravitate—Melville, Mimsy, Sasha, and Charcoal—but I could have. In the world of feline genetics, it's not off-base to see a link between color and temperament.

Geneticists who have traced the worldwide distribution of cats by coat color say the most common cat is the "blotched tabby"—the ones that are often called tigers—followed by black cats and, third, the red-headed league. The mutation that produces black cats "is linked through the hormonal system with a temperament that is less aggressive, less fearful, and more tolerant of crowding" than the wildcats from which they descend, writes the English specialist Dr. Juliet Clutton-Brock in *The British Museum Book of Cats.* The placid blotched tabby is a pussycat too, says Clutton-Brock, and these two types prevail in urban areas, where a mellow disposition has what Clutton-Brock calls "survival value."

But orange cats—which may have originated in Asia Minor and which are usually male (in females, the same gene produces calicos and tortoiseshells)—"have no particular survival value in large cities where they are never as common as black or blotched tabby cats," she writes.

No particular survival value. Reading between the lines, this enigmatic pronouncement hints that redheads like Tigger might have a genetic tendency to be, shall we say, high-strung—hotheads or scaredy-cats who don't do well in company. This characterization may or may not be true for anybody else's red cat, but as for mine, he was not what you would call laid-back.

It wasn't that Tigger was unfriendly. Quite the opposite; he liked people a lot. But he was far too jumpy to take full advantage of his own sociable impulses. Right after I got him, for example, I took him next door to visit Isabelle, where he sat for a while on an overstuffed armchair and stared at the birds flying in and out of her feeders like airplanes approaching O'Hare. Suddenly he got startled when one of us made a sudden movement, and dashed across the living room and into the kitchen, knocking over a couple of African violets as he run for cover. So much for convincing my neighbor, whose dog had recently died, that a kitten would make a good pet.

It was worse a few months later when he got into the Boans' place, next door to Isabelle's in the direction of the park.

Tigger liked to hang around the couple's front door and converse through the screen with their cat, Shadow, who is not allowed outside, and he became such a familiar guest that one day the Boans let him in. He picked his way through the kitchen as if it were a minefield, then got spooked and went reeling across the living room and dining room before hurling himself at the French doors and setting off the burglar alarm. Upon being told, I politely asked my neighbors to please not let Tigger in their house again.

On his own turf Tigger was more relaxed. He played with the big cats, and with me and any other humans who came around. And to my delight he proved to be something of a lap cat, curling up with me often and sometimes trying to "nurse" on my heavy alpaca wool sweater, as kittens taken too soon from their mothers will frequently do.

But he could be fretful, too. Sometimes when I picked him up he'd lean against me and purr. Other times he went rigid in my arms, twisted around to face me, and raised a paw as if he intended to slap. This happened most often when I caught him unawares and grabbed him from behind. It was defensive, not aggressive—Tigger's way of saying, *"Noli me tangere"*—but a little disconcerting nonetheless.

Unlike Sasha and Charcoal, who tend to be strong, silent types, Tigger talked a lot. He had something to say about everything, and sometimes stalked about muttering to himself under his breath. If I picked him up when he wasn't in the mood for it, he would respond with a cranky "Yow!"—kind of like "Meow" with the "Me" left off. It sounded a lot like "No!" and I soon deduced that was precisely what it meant. Another common utterance was the staccato "Eh-eh-eh-eh," which seemed to mean, "If you don't stop bothering me this instant I'm going to throw a fit." And sometimes he even would growl.

"He has issues," I would tell anyone who witnessed one of

these episodes, and I thought it likely that they stemmed from his early career as a street cat. If the boy who gave him to me was telling the truth, the kitten had once been abused, and there's no reason to think the same damage that occurs when humans are treated harshly doesn't also happen in young cats.

His excitable temperament, combined with sheer inexperience, made Tigger reckless once he got outdoor privileges. I began letting him out by himself when he was six or seven months old, and he found the freedom intoxicating. By now a rangy adolescent, long and lean as a greyhound, he was constantly getting into trouble.

One day he climbed thirty feet up the oak tree across the way and refused to come back down, mewing loudly until my neighbor Cory arrived with his tallest ladder to fetch him. Another time a friend leaned an aluminum ladder from my deck to the roof, a distance of two stories, in anticipation of doing some roof work for me. Working at my desk later that day, I happened to glance out the window to see, right at eye level, a stretch of fluffy, peach-colored tummy suspended between two rungs of the ladder. Rung by aluminum rung Tigger relentlessly climbed, and by the time I got outdoors he was already cavorting about on the roof, chasing leaves that had fallen on it. I'm a little bit afraid of heights, but I forced myself to follow him up the ladder and bring him down. This cat is too adventurous for his own good, I told myself; if he doesn't learn caution he'll have a short (but happy) life.

Sasha and Charcoal and I are attuned to one another's rhythms and adhere to a daily routine. I can usually count on them to be indoors every evening by 9:00 or 10:00 P.M.; nocturnal or not by nature, my cats aren't allowed to roam about all night. But Tigger didn't get with the program. The other two cats usually respond (albeit not always instantaneously) when I call their names, but not Tigger; and I spent more than one late night during the winter of Tigger's adolescence combing the neighborhood for him, boots on my feet and flashlight in hand. He would finally stagger in at eleven, midnight, 1:00 A.M., looking overwrought, haggard, and haunted—and then pass out like a toddler who has played too hard and too long. Where had he been? What had he done? Why hadn't he come when I called?

I got at least a partial answer one night when I stood by the front door in my parka with flashlight in hand and spotted a red cat racing down the road toward the house.

"Tigger!" I called, when suddenly from out of the shadows emerged another red cat racing along at the first one's heels. Tigger, it seemed, had found a friend—one who looked just like him, no less. On closer inspection, the strange cat's fur turned out to be a shade lighter than Tigg's, and his face a little rounder. But from a distance I couldn't tell them apart.

Like Sasha's pal Harlequin before him, this new red cat began hanging around the property after that. Also like Harlequin, he was skittish, and ran if I made the smallest move in his direction. He seemed uninterested in me, Sasha, Charcoal, or even in the food I left out for him once or twice, by which I deduced that he was not a stray but someone's roaming house cat. He was interested only in Tigger. Sometimes the two of them crouched nose to nose on the Boans' lawn and stared at each other, each looking tense and excited. Does a cat's sense of self extend to body image? Did Tigger know what he looked like—like Narcissus, did he see himself reflected in the face of this feline twin?

Whenever I tried to approach, the two cats would chase each other into the woods and out of my sight. Sometimes I heard them yowling, in a feline serenade not unlike Sasha's song to Buddy the day, years before, when the two of them discussed the rights of passage to Doris's lawn. And one night, in the depths of winter, Tigger and the red cat fought. I heard rather than saw it, a terrific caterwauling followed by a shriek of pain and a banging of the screen door; but when I opened it to let Tigger in, I found not my cat but only a couple of blood-stains and some tufts of fluffy red fur on the doorstep.

Tigger dragged himself home a half-hour later, frightened, bedraggled, and with an injured paw—a bite, it appeared—that later got infected and required a trip to the vet's. After that I curtailed his wanderings by refusing to let him out after 7:00 P.M., no matter how much he might stand by the door and complain. But as time went on I had the impression that Tigger grew grateful for the curfew. He relaxed, he became less edgy, and he seemed relieved that I was saving him from himself, so to speak. He sometimes saw the red cat during the day; merci-fully, I never saw evidence of another fight. But he spent the remainder of those long winter evenings curled up beside me on the couch.

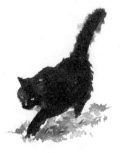

# 14  I Play, Therefore I Am

In the first snowfall of the first winter of the first year of his life, Tigger learned to dance.

Pausing for a moment at the workroom door to take in the strange state of the world outside, he stepped onto the whitened deck and shuffled across, like Jimmy Cagney doing a soft shoe in *Yankee Doodle Dandy*. He twirled, dove into the powder nose first to send it flying, then pawed it as it rained back down. He rolled around and around on his back and got up looking like a marzipan cat, liberally dusted with confectioner's sugar.

His joyfulness in motion made me think of the Shakers or the Dervishes, for whom to dance is to pray, and for a moment I had the feeling of being present at the Creation. Someone I respected once told me, "The Earth is God's laughter," and as I watched my red cat play I wondered if the Creator might not have a zesty sense of humor that He shares with all of his progeny, two-legged and four-legged alike.

There's nothing like having a kitten in the house to get you to think about play. Playing is a kitten's life, after all—I play, therefore I am. But no matter how familiar, it's a deeply mysterious subject. Play serves many functions and sometimes none. It can take the form of mock hunts or mock fights—rehearsals, or substitutes, for other behaviors. But it can also represent sheer high spirits, a way to kick up one's heels at the unparalleled joy of being alive. Witness Tigger's dance in the snow.

Another of the functions of play is to serve as a social glue, and this was a phenomenon I became acutely aware of as I watched Tigger's integration into the household. Play was the medium by which the kitten and the two black cats took one another's measure. Play let the juvenile get close to the adults in an exploratory way, and it gave him the physical contact with them that he seemed to crave. At the same time it reassured the big cats that although the little one might be a pest, he wasn't an enemy or challenger. He was just, well, playing.

The failure of Sasha's relationship with Mimsy and Jean Arthur had been, in essence, a failure of play. The two females never tolerated, appreciated, or even understood Sasha's attempts to draw them into play, for they interpreted his invitations as aggression.

Tigger was luckier. The black cats were both still playful themselves, younger and more physically robust than the two females had been when Sasha came to live with them. They were tolerant of the kitten's antics—especially when you consider how annoying he could be—and sometimes more than tolerant. If he got them in the right mood, Tigger could draw the other two into an enthusiastic romp and turn them into allies in the stalk, chase, and wrestle games he so enjoyed. He'll keep them young, I thought, or kill them trying.

First Tigger hit on Charcoal, whom he stalked and pounced upon fearlessly from the day he got out of quarantine. Poor Charcoal had a kitten draped around his neck more often than not in those days, and the naps he so cherished on his favorite blue-striped chair in front of the fireplace were no longer restful interludes. Tigger interrupted them with flying leaps and sneak attacks, and the only way Charcoal could get him to calm down was to pin him down with one paw and lick him thoroughly all over his head and face, just as a mother cat would. If it didn't quiet him down for long, this tactic succeeded in keeping the kitten immobile for at least as long as the bath took.

Tigger seemed to know instinctively that Charcoal was a pushover—or anyway, approachable. Of Sasha he was warier. For a while he quaked at the very sight of the top cat, ducking behind a piece of furniture when Sasha walked by, for example, or creeping under the bedroom bureau to sleep rather than risk approaching anywhere near the vicinity of Himself, asleep upon the bed.

Not that Sasha was particularly aggressive toward him. In fact, he wasn't all that interested in Tigger at first, and didn't interact with him much except to take an occasional, desultory sniff. Still, Tigger trembled when he realized Sasha was near, and if the top cat approached him—or sometimes just looked his way—Tigger instantly flung himself over on his side or rolled onto his back in order to expose his belly, body language that spoke submission.

Gradually Tigger's confidence grew, and he soon began approaching Sasha to play. He especially enjoyed sneaking up on the top cat outdoors, stalking him from some hiding place— behind the azalea, for example—and then rushing out at him.

Sasha would leap straight up in the air in surprise, then go streaking off into the bushes, with Tigger in eager pursuit.

Nevertheless, Sasha set limits whereas Charcoal did not, and for a very long time all he needed to do was to give Tigger the hairy eyeball and over on his back the red cat would roll, paws in the air and a "No offense—I was only fooling" expression on his face. Somehow, Tigger had assimilated the reality of Sasha's dominance and learned to respect it unquestioningly.

* * *

Researchers have found that humans are drawn to certain qualities in the animals we choose to live with, and playfulness is high among them. In general, it seems, we prefer animals that remind us of our own young—feisty, funny, and visually akin to a human baby, with large eyes and foreheads in a rounded face, like a pug dog or a Persian cat. This might explain the popularity of the Scottish fold, a newish breed of cat whose ears look like tiny kerchiefs folded snugly on its head. Seemingly earless, a fold's face is almost totally round, like a baby's or an owl's (strange, isn't it, how alike all we predators can look?).

We're suckers, in short, for the cute, the cuddly, and the playful—creatures who return our affection and look back at us with faces we can relate to as "one of ours." It's natural to be drawn to the familiar, after all, for what basis is there for understanding and acceptance—the cornerstones of love—if there is no common ground? Like attracts like, and maybe the only way to bridge the species gap is to see the animals we live with as more "like" than not. They do the same for us, anthropomorphism in reverse. Dogs, we are told, regard their human companions as fellow, albeit superior, dogs, dominant members of the pack. Cats are not pack animals in this same way, but they do grow up *en famille*, with a mother and siblings around. Perhaps my cats see me as the mom cat, giver of food, warmth, and comfort. But it seems more likely to me that they view me as an oversize, tailless litter mate; at any rate, they play with me as if I am. For it's not just cats and cats that learn to trust one another through play, it's cats and people, too. "When I play with my cat, how do I know that she is not passing time with me rather than I with her?" as Montaigne has it.

Tigger and I got to know each other in many ways, but playing was chief among them. I spent hours playing with my kitten, teasing him with the Cat Dancer, tempting him with a toy mouse or ball. His favorite toy was not man-made but a big wild-turkey feather I had picked up on a hike in the woods and displayed on a table, with assorted other found objects. Once Tigger discovered it, though, there was nothing to do but hand the feather over to him. I would trail it along the floor for him to chase and pounce upon, and he would grab it and run away as triumphantly as if he had downed the actual bird from which it came. By the time Tigger reached adolescence, this once noble plume was no more than a threadbare stalk. Ultimately I threw it away.

Even as grownups, my cats still like to engage me in play. When I walked upstairs from the workroom to the main floor of the house not long ago, for example, Sasha rushed out at me from his hiding place in the dining room and made a wide run around my ankles. He stopped short just out of my reach and looked back at me over his shoulder with mischief in his eyes. This was a signal that he wanted to play one of his favorite games: chase me.

I was up for it, and so I called out, "I'm going to get that cat! Where is he? Where's Sasha?" and made a pretend lunge in Sasha's direction that sent him flying onto one of the dining-room chairs. When I reached forward to poke at him through the tablecloth, a white-tipped paw emerged from under the lace, batting away like a manic metronome in its frenzy to nab me. I reached underneath, but the cat was too fast for me; he had already escaped to a different chair. (This game makes me think of one friend who believes cats don't realize they have tails. Like a very small child who thinks you can't see her when she's hiding her eyes, Sasha seemed to believe I wouldn't find him even though his bushy black tail lay draped over the edge of the chair, in plain sight.)

We moved around the table, from chair by chair, until Sasha emerged from under the cloth and made a mad dash for the living room, with me at his heels. He feinted left, tore around the couch, headed back toward the dining room. But to get there meant crossing my path, and before he could scoot by, I grabbed him. He wriggled free and hit the floor running, ready to do the circuit again and show me the true meaning of bop till you drop. Typically, I poop out of this game long before Sasha does.

In my house, other cat-initiated games include Let's tackle Jackie around the ankles and then pretend to run away and hide—ha ha ha; Newspaper (they bat at the page I'm on, sit atop the page I want to turn to next, or dive between the pages to make a crinkly paper tent); and Bathtub. Both Sasha and Tigger (but not Charcoal, who appears to be leery of the water) like to perch on the edge of the tub whenever I'm in it, pawing the running water or playing peekaboo games around the shower curtain. Another favorite game, of Tigger's, is to crouch at the top of the spiral staircase that connects the main house with the workroom downstairs, and tap me on the head when I climb it. He seems to get a boot out of being "taller" than I am for a change.

◆   ◆   ◆

Do cats have a sense of humor? To see Tigger's "Gotcha!" expression whenever he manages to nab me on the staircase, you might be tempted to say yes. But raising the question is risky, for it brings you to the metaphysical abyss called Consciousness, and the myriad arguments over who possesses consciousness and who does not. (I laugh, therefore I am?) What's more, it also requires coming up with a satisfactory definition of humor. At best that's a daunting task, at worst a hopeless one, for humor is elusive, subjective, evanescent, and bound, moreover, by cultural context. What's funny in the United States might not play in Botswana, Japan, or Brazil. Heck, even we English-speaking Americans don't always get British humor.

The "cultural context" for domestic cats rests in the fact that they live in our houses with us, so right away you've got a situation rich with comedic possibilities. Here we see shrewd predators, their skills perfected through millennia of natural selection, making themselves comfy in the unnatural environment of a human dwelling. Humor lies, at least in part, in the odd or ironic juxtaposition of unlike objects and events, and a cat indoors is as odd or ironic as you can get.

Take, for example, one universal feline activity: scratching sand (or litter) over his droppings to neatly cover them up. We think nothing of it when our cats do this at the litter box; it's part of what makes cats cats. Taken out of context, though, the gesture may well become a way of conveying humor.

One time my friend Linda and I were sitting in my living room having a snack—apple upside-down cake, I think it was—when Sasha leaped on the coffee table and bent down to sniff at my plate. Perhaps he was hoping for liver. He crinkled his nose in distaste and looked up at me knowingly. Then, without breaking eye contact, he began to scratch, his right paw moving incessantly back and forth across the glass top of the table, next to the dish. Scratching at the litter box is instinctive and comprehensible; but applied to apple upside-down cake, whatever could it mean?

A gustatory critique, was what I figured. "This is *merde* and deserves to be buried. How can you guys eat this stuff?"

Once you've come up with an interpretation, though, is there more to be said about intentionality? Could it be that Sasha was making a joke? It would be easier to join ranks with the skeptics—those who believe an animal's life is mechanical and deterministic—than to allow for the possibility that he was. Yet both Linda and I felt that afternoon that we were, in fact, being humorously mocked by a cat—that Sasha's action was neither random nor deterministic, but a considered reply to a particular stimulus. Using the only language available to him, that of feline behavior and biology, Sasha found a way to join our conversation on his own terms—even if all he had to utter was a rude remark. The wry, superior look on Sasha's face, and his clear expectation of raising a response, hint that maybe, just maybe, he thought he was being funny, too.

Catnip is another temptation to play. Some cats seem immune to the delights of this common herb—*Nepeta cataria,* according to the dictionary, a member of the mint family—but most of them find it irresistible. Ever since I planted a clump of catnip in my front garden, I get brownie points with my friends' cats by bringing them sprigs of the stuff (fresh in summer, dried in winter) when I visit. I myself have occasionally chomped one of the neat, serrated leaves in an attempt to discover what it is about this fragrant herb that causes the most staid and self-possessed of cats to caper about like a wind-up toy. I have yet to figure it out, though. The stuff doesn't do much for me. It tastes a little bit like peppermint: "bitter-aromatic, a bit strong, but not really unpleasant," in the words of the late herbalist Euel Gibbons, a champion of exotic edibles. Gibbons admitted to "almost constantly chewing catnip as I work around the yard and garden," but added, with some regret, that he didn't get as much fun out of the herb as his cat did.

The comedy in catnip lies in its ability to make a cat look

ridiculous. For although cats love to play, they deplore being made to look silly, unless it's on their own terms, i.e., I think I'll dive into a paper bag and run around the living room with it on my head. Cats don't mind if you laugh at them then, for they have chosen this gambit and are in control of it. (Plus, they like being the center of attention.) But if you're the one to put the paper bag on their heads, just watch how fast they squirm out of it and stalk off, all dirty looks and injured pride. If cats do have a sense of humor, it doesn't extend to being laughed at or laughing at themselves.

Cats are as image-conscious as a high-fashion model, and losing face is no joke. I suppose that's only fitting for a creature so elegant and urbane. To commit a gaffe or take an unintended pratfall must seem, to a cat, akin to a prima ballerina tripping on pointe and tumbling to the stage in a heap of tulle. The hypothetical dancer might pick herself up, dust off her tutu, and go on with the show. What a cat does is to begin grooming compulsively, as if to say, "Nothing happened—really! I'm just sitting here washing my paws over and over again, which is what I intended to do all along. Don't give it another thought!" Displacement behavior, it's called. You can make a cat truly miserable by laughing at a time like this.

All cats are particular about losing face, but some are more sensitive to it than others. The status-conscious Sasha is quick to take offense—he finds no solace in the old saw, "I'm laughing *with* you, not *at* you"—while Charcoal and Tigger remain comparatively unruffled. My friends' old gray cat Nigel, who was none too bright even in his salad days, usually failed to notice when he was being laughed at. However, even he was thoroughly shamefaced the day his owners caught him creeping stealthily forward to assess the threat posed by the stalking-cat garden ornament that had just been installed in the front yard.

The very fact that cats can't bear being laughed at when

they're caught doing something awkward, unintended, or foolish makes it hard not to. It's an unfortunate aspect of human
nature, perhaps, that we're not above finding humor in some-
body else's misfortunes. Who among us can resist laughing
when we see some fool slip on the proverbial banana peel? (And
who among us wants to be the fool who takes the fall?)

The other day, for example, Sasha was fast asleep on the
arm of the couch when all of a sudden he fell off, awakening in
wide-eyed confusion at having plunged so ignominiously to the
floor. It was hard not to laugh at the sight of such a self-assured
creature so thoroughly and uncharacteristically befuddled. But
since I'm well aware of Sasha's sensitivity in this regard, I
managed to stifle, more or less successfully, my mirth. Sasha
immediately began washing his face with more than the usual
meticulousness. Then, having recovered his aplomb, he stalked
off to the bedroom in a show of dignity regained. Presumably,
he found a safer spot there to nap.

Sometimes I'm less able to suppress a laugh, however.
Sasha is a great jumper, and he seems to take pride in his ability
to vault, in seemingly effortless leaps, to the highest points in
the house—eight feet to the top of the corner cupboard in the
living room, for instance, where he curls up to sleep in the big
basket I keep up there. Even with a table nearby to use as a
springboard, such a jump requires both athletic ability and a
grasp of elementary physics. A miscalculation of height or trajectory can result in a misstep, a rude tumble instead of a graceful ascent.

One night not long ago just such a blunder occurred, and
Sasha missed the top of the cupboard by several crucial inches.
He slid awkwardly down its sides, grasping at each of the lower
shelves as he passed them in a vain attempt to break his fall. He
landed with a thud.

Whether he was shaken by the gross indignity of the episode or humiliated by the fact that I couldn't help laughing, he gave himself only a few cursory grooming licks before heading for the door. Apparently, removing himself from the scene of the debacle was the only way to repair his tarnished ego.

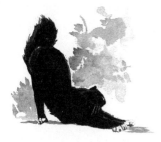

# 15  Copycat

It's been my observation that kittens raised with other cats are better adjusted, and just plain *nicer*, than kittens raised by their human companions alone. I don't have hard evidence to back this up. It's just an impression, bolstered by the haphazard example of assorted cats I've know who were rescued young and grew up around no one but people. These cats don't know how to do things that cats ordinarily can do. Drink, for instance. One friend found his cat, whom he named Itty for her diminutive size, when she was just two or three weeks old, and fed her with an eyedropper until she could manage to eat by herself. But she never got the hang of water. She plunks her nose in the bowl, then comes up confusedly for air and sneezes a big watery sneeze. She much prefers drinking from the tap or from the hose that bubbles into the fish tank.

Itty went through a rambunctious stage, as kittens do, but in her case it's lasted and lasted. My friend is a patient man. He was adept at calming her down whenever she started bouncing off the walls like a Nerf ball. He stayed cool as she heated up, and usually succeeded in getting her behavior back within normal kittenish bounds (not out of Emily Post in the best of cases).

But without other cats around to teach her good manners the feline way, this little tiger can still be a terror at almost a year—except that now she's fully equipped with fangs and grownup, feline claws. If left to her own devices, she uproots potted plants and eats angel fish right out of the aquarium. My friend is hoping that a handsome white and black cat named Visitor, an exceedingly well-mannered individual who has just joined the household, will be a good influence on her.

Tigger didn't have Itty's problem, of course, for he grew up under the tutelage of two adult male cats, who together taught him the rules of the road and socialized him to the ways of the household. He was a young, inexperienced cat, and he looked to them for cues. It was a subtle process. But over time I came to see that Tigger was learning what was expected of him, what behaviors were allowable, by the feline example he saw before him.

When the eminent zoologist George B. Schaller did field-work for his classic study of East African lions, he took note of the fascination cubs seemed to have for the males of the pride. "From a cub's point of view, males must be surly brutes, for most attempts to draw them into play are rebuffed with a slap or growl," Schaller wrote in *Golden Shadows, Flying Hooves*, his 1973 memoir of his work in Tanzania. "Yet cubs are strangely drawn to these strong and withdrawn members of the pride.

They like to sit by males and imitate them by, for example, yawning or sharpening claws when they do."

So it was with Tigger.

Tigger followed the black cats around. He sat with them, napped when they did, ate when they did. He constantly monitored what they were doing, and over and over I watched him begin to take some action—lie down on the living-room rug, for example—and then change his mind when he saw that the other two cats were doing something different; heading upstairs, say, to nap in the bedroom. Upstairs, then, Tigger too would go.

Sasha and Charcoal introduced him to the pleasures of the fireplace, in front of which the cats would lounge that first winter in threes or in twos. They taught him the etiquette of dining: namely, Sasha eats from the bowl on the left and Charcoal from the one on the right, which meant Tigger should eat in the middle. He dogged Sasha's footsteps outdoors, and it was my impression that he initially learned his way around the neighborhood—the territorial boundaries—this way. And he learned by the black cats' example to quash his inclination to wake me up in the wee hours, as he tried to do when he first joined the household. In my house, cats, like people, wait until the alarm clock goes off, and after a while Tigger adopted this habit too.

When spring arrived, the young cat began to hunt. He proved to be a quick study, and soon was bringing his catches home, not to me but to whichever of the black cats happened to be around at the time. I once watched him pop out of the hedges with a bird in his mouth and canter over to the side garden to lay it down in front of Sasha, as if for approval. Together the two cats admired the corpse for a good long while, walking all about it like car buyers examining a Miata and pawing it every so often, perhaps to make sure it was dead.

It's hard for a kitten, as for a child, to learn to control his own impulses, but Sasha and Charcoal helped Tigger in this regard by supplying external discipline to compensate for the lack of inner controls—usually when he was carried away by the intensity of his play. If pinning him down and washing his face didn't help, Charcoal's first line of defense, a smack in the head, might do it. Like old-fashioned schoolteachers who believed sparing the rod meant spoiling the child, the black cats were not above giving Tigger a good clout when he got out of line.

But they watched out for him, too. Charcoal, especially, often bathed Tigger and invited him up for naps *à deux* on Charcoal's favorite chair. And Sasha seemed to welcome the kitten's company outdoors, now that Charcoal, his erstwhile companion, had largely lost his appetite for adventure. The relationships were fluid, not static; ever-shifting alliances as the grown cats allowed the young one in and the three animals cemented their friendship.

*   *   *

By the time that Tigger showed up, Sasha and Charcoal had been living together for almost six years. They had grown accustomed—indeed, preternaturally attuned—to each other, as a series of photographs taken not long before Tigger's arrival reminded me. Perhaps because I'm not a very good photographer and can't ever seem to get the image I want, I tend to waste a lot of film on my cats. As a result, I have a whole drawer full of blurry, out-of-focus prints. This one roll, however, contained three rather extraordinary shots.

In the first picture, Sasha and Charcoal are perched on the little wooden shelf I installed for them under the front living-room window, which lacks a windowsill big enough for cats. They are sitting at attention, one on either side of the shelf, like bookends. Two black tails—one sleek as an eel, one fluffy as a feather duster—arc gracefully over the edge. Sasha turns his head to face the camera and Charcoal, his *doppelgänger*, turns the other way, facing out.

In the second shot, the cats are curled up asleep on the bed, nestled against each other in a double parenthesis amid a mound of comforters.

In the third picture, they are standing on top of the TV. Sasha is in the foreground heading north, Charcoal is behind him angled south, but their postures are otherwise identical, and both cats cock their heads sideways to stare at the camera. The foreshortening is such that together they appear to make a two-headed cat—a feline version of Dr. Dolittle's push-me, pull-you.

It's not by chance that I happened to get these three shots on a single roll of film. The longer Sasha and Charcoal lived together, I found, the more they took to settling into identical or mirror-image poses, apparently quite unconsciously but always with the utmost grace and fluidity of motion. It was as if some inner choreographer were directing a subtle, two-way pantomime: Let's pose in front of the fireplace like the recumbent stone lions in front of the New York Public Library. Let's sit up on our haunches, straight and tall, like Egyptian cat statues. Let's curl up on the comfortable new chair in the living room, head to head and tail to tail, with our backs arced symmetrically against its abundantly upholstered arms.

It's almost spooky to come upon cats when they're engaged in these tableaux vivants. Is this some otherworldly ritual, the meaning of which mere humans can never fathom? Or could it be that cats really are aesthetes, as some of us have long suspected? Symmetrical and contrapuntal movements, after all, are the stuff of dance and of art. Two cats posed in harmonic juxtaposition make a more pleasing picture than two cats reclining at random.

Aesthetics aside, it seems safer to assume that cats who live together, like Sasha and Charcoal, must be deeply influenced by one another's presence. So much so, perhaps, that they gradually absorb each other's emotional or attitudinal coloration, subtly growing to more closely resemble each other in style and manner, the way that siblings sometimes do, or couples who have been married a long time. They also borrow from each other's behavioral repertoire, as I came to see when Charcoal first joined the household and began copying things that Sasha would do.

For example, Sasha is in the habit of bounding grandly, claws extended, onto the topmost panel of the screen door whenever he wants to come in. This invariably causes a stir. The clatter of the rattling door and the sight of the cat self-importantly defying gravity upon it makes for a grand entrance. One visiting child was so impressed that he vowed to train his own cat to do the same thing, until his father pointed out that their Brooklyn brownstone lacks one essential ingredient: a screen door.

One summer night I heard the shake, rattle, and roll of the screen door, but when I went to see who was there I found it was Charcoal, not Sasha. He's not the cat he used to be before the shooting incident in which his back left leg was injured—it stole some of his agility, and he runs with the whisper of a limp—so he couldn't levitate to the top of the screen, six feet off the ground, the way that Sasha does. Instead he was half-standing, half-hanging at the door, his front claws resolutely gripping its bottom panel as he groped for a toehold on the narrow doorjamb. On Charcoal's face was an expression that mixed embarrassment with elation. He wasn't quite sure if he should be proud of himself, but he wanted to be.

After first becoming aware that Charcoal had copycat aspirations, I soon began to notice them often. Sasha liked to jump on the hood of the car when I first pulled into the driveway (leaving muddy paw prints all over it). Now Charcoal began to do it, too. Sasha would scratch at the drawer of the bureau in the bedroom so that I'd open it, allowing him to settle down for a nap amid my sweaters. Charcoal followed him in. Sasha then demanded that the cedar chest be opened so he could curl up there instead. Upon reflection, Charcoal found himself agreeing that the cedar chest was a much better spot for a nap than the sweater drawer, and he jumped out of the one to join his pal in the other.

Sasha likes to patrol the narrow shelf that's built along the length of the loft bedroom's balconylike half-wall, from which he can look down into the living room like an eagle on a cliff. One night Charcoal jumped up there too, but he chose the worst possible section of it for his maiden voyage. Instead of the relatively uncluttered central portion where Sasha always goes, he squeezed his seventeen pounds into the farthest right-hand corner, where there's precious little head room thanks to the house's sloping eaves, and precious little lateral room because of the books I've tucked into that space.

Fearful that the Oxford illustrated edition of the complete works of Jane Austen would come crashing to the floor, I lifted the cat away. He looked somewhat relieved and a little befuddled, as if he couldn't understand why his foray was met with consternation while the other cat's shelf prowling is not.

❖ ❖ ❖

We live in a culture that prizes individualism and prosecutes plagiarists. But objectively speaking, there's nothing intrinsically wrong with copying the example of another (or even, sometimes, his work, as in the long tradition of folk music, where successive generations put new lyrics to old tunes). Imitation is the sincerest form of flattery—possibly even of love, or at least affiliation. Members of any peer group use jargon that serves to link them even as it excludes others, be they electrical engineers talking RAMS and ROMS or the Crips and the Bloods talking street talk. They may dress alike, too, *The Wild Ones* in motorcycle jackets, the Generation Xers in Doc Martens, and the nerds from all those *Far Side* cartoons in white shirts with pocket protectors.

Closer to home, children mimic their parents and others in their circle as they grope toward a definition of self, and this is no less true in animal societies than human ones. Far from betraying a lack of imagination, the ability to copy the example of one's mentors, and to practice techniques they might show us, is a sign of intelligent life.

I never saw Beanhead, the mother cat of my childhood, teach her kittens to hunt, as cats are reported to do. But I did watch her instruct them in another feline art form: tree climbing. Bean would scale the huge ash tree that rose over our backyard like the mast of a great ship, with a kitten or two at her heels; then stop short two thirds of the way up. She would deliberately begin backing down, hindquarters first, which forced the kittens to do likewise, and mother and children would soon find themselves descending all the way to solid ground. *Voilà!* The descent demystified.

This very valuable lesson is one that some cats never learn. My cat Mimsy was one of them, despite having come of age in a multi-cat household alongside her mother and siblings. Mimsy could climb a tree all right, but she didn't know what to do once she had. She'd either mew pitifully until someone came and got her, or maneuver around on a branch in order to head down the trunk the same way she went up: nose first. She would inevitably gain speed and lose her grip as she made this precipitous descent, and land with a big awkward thump.

But there's copying and there's copying. As Tigger got bigger, I began to notice that while he mimicked the example of both black cats in a general way, he was beginning to single out Sasha for specific emulation, just as Charcoal had before him. But where Charcoal had simply picked up a few tricks from a feline model he seemed to admire—one who preceded him in the household and thus knew its manners and mores—Tigger appeared to have another agenda. As if out of a textbook of Freudian psychology, this young prince suddenly seemed to covet what the king possessed.

The surest way to attain status, I suppose, is to usurp someone else's, and I started feeling a bit sorry for Sasha as Tigger, around the time of his first birthday, began to test him. It can't be any picnic being top cat, for the leader by definition is the one to beat, and Sasha now found himself in the position of a veteran gunslinger challenged by a cocky young cowpoke. For example, Sasha often demands that things that are closed be opened for him, and one day he began scratching at a covered basket I keep in the bedroom. I obliged by raising the lid and removing a couple of items stashed inside so as to make room for him to jump in it.

Tigger had never expressed interest in this basket before, but now that Sasha had imbued it with significance, the young cat suddenly found the basket intensely attractive. As Sasha did the obligatory circling around in preparation for lying down to sleep, Tigger approached the basket. Head held high, his body language seeming to bristle, he fixed his copper gaze on Sasha in an attitude of bald challenge.

Sasha registered immediately that this was a test. He jumped out of the basket and on top of the red cat, who at this point was no kitten but a sleek, muscular young tom weighing in at twelve pounds—two pounds more than Sasha himself. The two began to tussle, rolling around on the rug in a heap of black and orange, yipping, and nipping at each other's paws and throats in another of the strange, formalized wrestling matches I've become accustomed to since Sasha came to live with me. As ferocious as these encounters sometimes look, there is a ritualized quality to them that differentiates them from true catfights, which can be appalling, and even deadly.

Tigger abruptly tore away from Sasha's clinch to fling himself over on his side in submission. Nothing overt had happened to tilt the battle in Sasha's direction. But it must have been unnerving (albeit thrilling) to tussle with the alpha cat this way, and I imagine Tigger must have sensed he was pushing Sasha's patience a little beyond the tolerable. He rolled over onto his back and waved his paws in the air: "I yield!" Satisfied, Sasha turned his back on the youngster and headed again toward the basket.

But Tigger would not let it go. He crept toward the basket again, following a step or two behind Sasha. But by now he was losing his nerve. In contrast to the cocky attitude that marked his first approach, this time he sidled up to the top cat with head held low—and backed off instantly as soon as Sasha feinted a move in his direction. The response sent Tigger dancing across the room sideways, on tiptoe. He plunked himself down on the rug, stomach exposed, and stared as Sasha got into the basket one more time.

Foolish Tigger—he couldn't keep away. No sooner had Sasha begun to settle in than Tigger approached once more; but this time he turned tail and ran down the stairs the instant Sasha raised his head above the basket's rim and gave him a dirty look. Somehow, Sasha had conveyed the message that he would tolerate no more testing. With the challenger finally vanquished, he settled down in the basket for a hard-earned snooze.

Apparently, though, longings for the basket weighed on Tigger's mind. Just as a cookie jar once owned by Andy Warhol

is vastly more coveted by collectors than one owned by you or
me, so Sasha's acquisition of the basket had suffused this hum-
ble object with an irresistible allure. When he vacated it later in
the day to go outside, Tigger crept back upstairs. And when I
went up to get something out of the bedroom, guess who I
found in the basket?

Tigger stood in it upright (did he fear that if he let down
his guard, Sasha might catch him unawares?), looking as smug
and complacent as the proverbial cat who has just eaten the ca-
nary. The simple act of occupying a spot the top cat had
deemed desirable seemed to give Tigger immense satisfaction.
He had raised his status in his own eyes, and judging by his
expression, it sure felt good.

Tigger got to sleep in the basket that night as Sasha—now
uninterested in this prize, and seemingly unaware of the triumph it represented for the red cat—assumed his usual spot on
the bed. In fact, after that incident, Sasha never bothered with
the basket again, though whether this was due to Tigger's ap-
propriating it or simple lack of interest I cannot tell; it's as if the
basket simply vanished from Sasha's mental landscape. As for
Charcoal, he never had basket-envy. At seventeen pounds he's
much too big to get into it, and he snoozed in a favorite spot
atop the cedar chest throughout the other cats' tussle.

The basket looms large in Tigger's emotional life to this
day. Having managed to lay claim to this hallowed ground, he
took to sleeping in it frequently, and by now it is pretty much
his. I don't even attempt to close the lid any more; it sits perma-
nently open, and there's nothing inside but a pair of old wool
leg warmers that I tucked in to make my cat a bed.

"Where's Tigger?" asked a friend who came over the other
night.

"Probably upstairs in his basket," I said, the fact of owner-
ship now firmly established.

The power struggles in the household have diminished as Tigger has grown, and today the three cats reside in a reasonably stable firmament. Sasha remains the North Star; he succeeded in fighting off any threat to his dominance that Tigger might have posed, and all three cats appear happier for having defined and solidified the parameters of their roles. While those roles do involve acquiescence to a leader, the concept of hierarchy goes just so far. Sasha is top cat, it is true, but neither of the other two is "bottom" cat. There's only "not top cat" and "also not top cat."

Thanks to their long association, Sasha and Charcoal are closer to each other than either of them is to Tigger. They usually sleep side by side at the foot of the bed, for example, while Tigger sleeps on the other side of the queen-size mattress—or in his much loved basket, at the foot. But all three cats share an easy camaraderie; they all seem to, well, *like* each other.

Tigger will never be mellow—I watched aghast as he pranced merrily about Isabelle's steeply pitched roof just the other day—but he is a calmer cat than I feared he might grow up to be, and I owe that to Sasha and Charcoal. Any worries I had that three cats are one cat too many have long since been put to rest.

# Acknowledgments

This book would not have been written without a little help from my friends. Linda Epstein Dickey was central, for it was she who instructed me to "write a book about Sasha," and she who served as first reader for virtually everything between these covers. I am grateful for her generosity of spirit as well as for her insights and editorial suggestions.

I likewise owe a debt of gratitude to another early reader, Susan Dwyer Metzger. Her faith in the book sustained me, and her enthusiasm was crucial to its publication, for it was Susan who played matchmaker between me and my publisher, W. W. Norton.

For moral support and hand-holding during the time I was

writing, I relied especially on the kindness and good humor of George Borecky III, as well as Patricia Bayer, Susan Bronson, Lisa Iarkowski, my brother, Michael T. Damian, and my mother, Norma Damian.

Cat (and dog) stories came from near and far, with a few even arriving on-line from CompuServe subscribers who kindly allowed me to quote from their musings on scoopable litter. They are Martha Ashley, Helen Karbe, Janet McConnaughey, Gayle Sanders, Lorraine Shelton, and David Towle.

Closer to home, Ann Courchaine, Beth Eastman and Ben Eichler, Doris Cox Foos, Karen Gaudette, Greg Lupion, Stan and Nora Metzger, Cliff Post, Eleanore Speert, Joanne Taylor, and Howard Wolff are among those who offered insights, anecdotes, and encouragement.

I thank my editor, Carol Houck Smith, for making me sharpen my writing and clarify my thoughts. This is a better book than it would have been without her.

My very special thanks go to George and Claudette Field, who believed in this project long before there was any reason to, and to Dr. Alice Maher, who gave me the confidence to begin.

Finally, I'd also like to thank Dr. Richie Dubensky, Carol Ladwig, and Barbara Miller at the Milford Animal Hospital for taking such good care of my cats.